Healthy by *Design*

Get Active, God's Way

Weight Loss Devotional
and Workout Challenge

Lose weight, learn to love exercise,
and glorify God with your body

Cathy Morenzie

Guiding Light Publishing

Published: July 2020

ISBN: 978-1-9992207-6-1 (print)
978-1-9992207-7-8 (digital)

Published by Guiding Light Publishing
46 Bell St. Barrie ON Canada L4N 0H9

Note: The information in this book is for educational purposes only and is not recommended as a means of diagnosing or treating illness. All situations concerning physical or mental health should be supervised by a health professional knowledgeable in treating that particular condition. Neither the author nor anyone affiliated with Healthy by Design dispenses medical advice, nor do they prescribe any remedies or assume any responsibility for anyone who chooses to treat themselves.

Cover & author photos by martinbrownphotography.com

Interior Design by: Davor Dramikanin

Table of Contents

A Note From the Author

I want you to imagine your gym clothes folded and set out in a nice little pile at the foot of your bed. As your eyes pop open in the morning, without giving it a second thought you jump into your clothes and head out the door for your morning walk. As you walk, as you take in the morning sights, as you hear the birds singing and smell the fresh morning dew, as you breathe in the fresh air, as your body effortlessly allows you to walk and for all that awaits you today, do you give thanks for it all?

If you can't even fathom that morning scenario, imagine this... It's twelve noon and your day is already piling up. You've got phone calls to return, deadlines to meet, you feel tired and lack energy, yet without giving it a second thought you drop what you're doing and get in your daily dose of exercise. And to top it off, because of your renewed energy you're able to effectively tend to all of the other tasks you laid aside to make time for exercise.

Sound like crazy talk?

What if I told you that this could be you by next month?

If this still sounds like something out of a work of fiction, then this book is for you.

Although I've been in the exercise field for all of my adult life, exercise did not ever come naturally to me unless I was getting paid to lead a class. However, over the years I've learned to make physical activity part of my daily routine.

I wish I could tell you that I love exercise and I can't wait to do it each day, but that would be a lie. Truth is, I don't have any emotional attachment to exercise. I just wake up every day and do it. I don't ask myself if I should do it or not, I don't check the weather forecast to determine whether I will exercise today, and I don't beat myself up if I don't do it. It's just a way of life for me—as natural as eating, brushing my teeth, or taking a shower. It is now a routine and a way of life.

And although exercise is a great weight-releasing tool, I no longer see it as a form of punishment for when I overeat or solely as a way to burn fat, like I used to in the past.

Exercise for me is worship!

It's time that I spend with the Lord, giving Him glory and thanks for the ability to move. It's my time where I crank up my worship music and give Him praise, or it may be a more solemn time where I reflect on the coming days or simply get focused by dedicating my day to God.

Making exercise a daily habit was a matter of changing the way I perceived it. Understanding how important it was, not only for my health but also for my mental, emotional and spiritual health, too.

Transforming the way you think about exercise so it can become part of your daily routine is possible for you, too, my friend, but it won't happen by just wishing or wanting. And it's not about trying to encourage yourself with slogans like 'Just do it' or 'just trust God'. That will only end in frustration, guilt, and disappointment yet again. Best part is, you don't have to waste years trying to figure out how to make yourself do it.

By the end of this book you will gain an entirely new perspective on exercise— one that you may have never imagined was possible.

You will shift your focus from seeing exercise as a painful chore to something that is part of your everyday routine.

To give you a head start, I'm offering you these special gifts just for purchasing this book:

Enjoy three getting-started workouts to help you kickstart your journey: These simple, easy-to-follow workouts are designed to safely shape and tone every body part, while stretching your muscles to decrease your chances of injury.

Plus you'll receive my *Three Steps to Overcoming Emotional Eating* guide and our insightful, honest, and inspiring emails on all things related to weight loss, God's way.

weightlossgodswaybonus.com

What to expect as you read this book

I'm an avid reader.

This allows me to appreciate books from both vantage points. As a reader, I appreciate knowing ahead of time what I can expect so that I can manage my expectations and pace myself for what is to come.

Expect Resistance

I'll be the first to admit that I've stopped reading books when the material was 'hard', or it started ruffling my feathers. I know it's good for me, but my flesh was not prepared to receive it. So now you're sufficiently forewarned. You may experience resistance as you read this book. Resistance is push-back from yourself that you will feel. It is part of the process of growth and change. Don't be surprised when it comes. Some resistance is God perfecting us, and some is the enemy keeping us from our victory. Discern which is which, and exercise the power of prayer accordingly.

Yes, you may want to quit. Yes, the enemy will try to convince you that you can't do it. Know that victory is waiting on the other side.

"Consider it pure joy, my brothers and sisters, whenever you face trials of many kinds because you know that the testing of your faith produces perseverance. Let perseverance finish its work so that you may be mature and complete, not lacking anything." (Jas. 1:2-4)

Expect to Work

You will get out of this book exactly what you put in. If you don't do the work then you cannot expect to see a change.

I also suggest that you put the principles into place by challenging yourself to participate in some type of physical activity each day.

Choose your level:

Level 1 - Not currently exercising at all. Your goal is to begin moving for at least five minutes per day.

Level 2 - Exercising every once in a while, but not consistently. Your goal is to move consistently each day for at least 15 minutes.

Level 3 - Exercising consistently and ready to up your game. Your goal is to exercise each day for at least 30 minutes.

"Whatever you do, work at it with all your heart, as working for the Lord, not for men, since you know that you will receive an inheritance from the Lord as a reward. It is the Lord Christ you are serving." (Col. 3:23-25)

Expect Renewed Joy and Hope in the Lord

Something beautiful begins to happen when you spend more time with the Lord. He will minister to your heart and soul. Expect that your relationship with the Lord will be strengthened as a result of this journey.

Expect to Feel Fear

Fear is at the root of most of the things that stop us in life. As you read this book, all kinds of fears may come out of the woodwork. Fear of injury, fear of failure, fear of commitment. Just be aware of them and know that, in due season, they will be dealt with. Resist the urge to try to confront too many fears at once. Just know that it exists, and resist the urge to run and hide when you experience it.

Expect Changes in your Patterns

Are you always doing things at the last minute, then wondering why things don't work out for you?

Maybe you do not take the time to plan when you will exercise. There will be habits that you notice that will get in the way of your success—journal them and turn them over to the Lord. You can't change everything at once, but you should make note of it for future reference.

How to use this book

I suggest you read through the 28 days of the devotional, one day at a time.

The goal is to allow God to change you from the inside out. This is a process, and it takes time. If you rush through it, you will miss the gold that God has for you in the pages of this book.

Most of the 28 days contains six sections: scripture reflection, devotion, reflect, pray, my prayer, and additional scriptures.

Below are some instructions on how to use each of these sections. Don't feel like you need to do all of them each day.

Scripture Reflection:

"Oh, how I love your law!
I meditate on it all day long."
(Psalm 119:97)

Study the daily scripture as you go about your day.

Write it down, ask the Holy Spirit to bring it to your remembrance when appropriate. Put it on your fridge or on the dashboard of your car—anywhere you will be able to refer to it a few times a day. It's the Word of God that has the power to change us to meditate on His word.

Devotion:

*"So we have come to know and to believe the love
that God has for us. God is love, and whoever abides
in love abides in God, and God abides in him."*
(1 John 4:16)

The devotion introduces the main topic in both a practical and spiritual context. Read it to understand how the Holy Spirit is leading and guiding you. Each devotion is designed to bring you back to the overarching truth, that God is calling you to rise up and take action, and He promises to be with you on your journey.

Reflect:

Life can get so busy. Even our devotion time can become something else to do on our to-do list. Taking time to reflect allows us to slow down and think about how the daily topics affect you and your relationship with God. The daily reflection will give you a better understanding of yourself in light of the Word of God. Read the questions at the start of the day and reflect on them throughout the day.

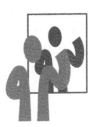

Pray:

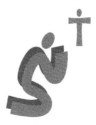

Enjoy the daily guided prayer. Sometimes it can be difficult to articulate what's in your heart, so I've provided you with guided prayers that you can make your own to cry out to God.

Each prayer is a beautiful summary of the daily scripture and devotion.

My Prayer:

In addition to the guided prayer, I encourage you to take some time and journal your personal prayers to God, sharing your heart with Him. Pour your heart out to God. Speak His Word back to Him; confess, declare, supplicate, and cry out to Him in prayer. James 5:16 teaches us that the prayer of a righteous person is powerful and effective.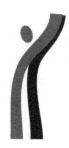

Additional Scriptures:

I've included some additional scriptures at the end of each day if you want to delve deeper into the topic. God's Word is so rich and powerful. The more you study His Word the greater your insight will become.

Ready? Let's go!

Devotional

Day 1:
Why RISE UP?

Scripture Reflection

> *Jesus said to him, "Rise, take up your bed and walk."*
> *(John 5:8 KJV)*

Devotion

There's a story in the Bible of a man who had been infirm for 38 years. Jesus finds him waiting by the pool called Bethesda, waiting for miraculous healing. *"Jesus asks him, 'Do you want to get well?' The man replies, 'Sir, I have no man to put me into the pool when the water is stirred up; but while I am coming, another steps down before me.' (John 5:1-8)*

Without missing a beat, Jesus tells him, *"Rise, take up your bed and walk."* Immediately the man was made well and took up his bed and walked.

There's so much we can learn from this story and apply our own challenges to getting more active and healthy. We may not be paralyzed, but we've been struggling for many, many years with strongholds that have kept us bound. Like the infirm man, we've held on to the belief that we have no one to help us. That we're alone. That we will never be free from the bondage. We, too, have been stuck.

Like the infirm man, you may also have found yourself talking more about your struggles than the success you want to achieve. You may become so consumed by your current circumstances that you don't believe that you can ever get well. And like him, your excuses may be bigger than your expectations.

Jesus' command to him was simple, clear, and direct—"RISE!" There were no justifications, rationalizations, or questions. There was no need to address his fears or excuses—just a command to "RISE!", followed by "take up your mat and walk." Jesus was calling for action.

We learn that the man was waiting by the pool because he believed that his healing would come from the 'magic waters', but Jesus showed him another way. A better way. One that did not require him to fight to be first in line or that would require others to help him. Jesus healed him by the simple command, "RISE UP!"

Upon Jesus' directive, the man began walking. As you read this, can you hear Jesus extending the same opportunity to you?

- It's time to let go of what's been holding you back and RISE UP!

- It's time to stop believing in magic potions and lotions and trust God for your victory.

- It's time to walk out of your place of discomfort, discouragement, depression, and despair and do what God says to do.

IT'S TIME TO RISE UP!

As you read this book and challenge yourself to get active, let this be your rally cry each day. Hear Jesus encouraging you to rise up! Throughout this book, you will be studying this passage in great detail as you challenge yourself to make exercise part of your daily routine.

Be encouraged as you read the daily devotions. Participate in the daily challenge, trusting and believing that God has transformed you from the inside out. You are a new creation in Him (2 Col. 5:17).

Reflect

As it relates to getting active, how is the Holy Spirit calling you to let go of what's been holding you back and RISE UP?

_____

_____

_____

_____

_____

Why is it important for you to Rise Up in this season of your life?

_____

_____

_____

_____

_____

As you read John 5:8, what do you hear the Holy Spirit calling you to do?

_____

_____

_____

_____

_____

Pray

Dear Lord, I'm about to embark on another journey and it's one that has kept me bound for such a long time. Here I go, Lord. You know my fears, You know my schedule, and You know what keeps holding me back from truly rising up and embracing exercise fully. So I turn this process over to You and I lay it at Your feet.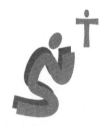
Give me a healthy perspective on exercise. One that does not include pain, punishment or self-gratification, but one that is based on glorifying You and You alone, by the end of this devotional challenge. Allow me to put exercise in its rightful place in my everyday life. I give You my body today as my reasonable service to You. In Jesus' Name, amen!

My Prayer

_____

_____

_____

_____

_____

_____

_____

Additional Scriptures

"But that ye may know that the Son of man hath power on Earth to forgive sins, (then saith he to the sick of the palsy,) Arise, take up thy bed, and go unto thine house".
(Matthew 9:6 NIV)

"Then will the lame leap like a deer, and the mute tongue shout for joy. Water will gush forth in the wilderness and streams in the desert." (Isaiah 35:6 NIV)

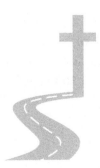

Day 2:

Exercise 101

Scripture Reflection

"She dresses herself with strength and makes her arms strong."
(Proverbs 31:17 ESV)

Devotion

Exercise conjures up different thoughts for different people. For some people, it means going to a gym and pumping iron. For others, it means sweating and painful muscles, while for others, it's a relaxing walk with a friend. They are all forms of exercise.

Today, you will understand exactly what exercise is and learn all of the necessary components that you need to incorporate into a well-rounded exercise routine.

Exercise can be defined as simply any bodily activity or movement that enhances or maintains physical fitness and overall health and wellness. Based on this definition, it can include anything from dancing to gardening.

However, a well-rounded fitness program involves three components: cardiovascular fitness, muscular strength, and flexibility.

The activities you choose to incorporate into your fitness regime will be based on your goals and personal preferences. To maximize fat loss, you will probably need to increase the amount of time you spend performing both cardiovascular and muscular conditioning or strength training.

Here is a detailed description of the three components:

Cardiovascular Fitness (or aerobic exercise)

Is the ability of your heart and lungs to supply oxygen-rich blood to all the muscles in the body. It is strengthened by performing activities such as running, walking, swimming, cycling, or anything that will elevate your heart rate.

Benefits:

1. Improves cardiovascular health
2. Lowers blood pressure
3. Helps regulate blood sugar
4. Reduces asthma symptoms
5. Reduces chronic pain
6. Aids sleep
7. Regulates weight
8. Strengthens immune system
9. Improves brain power
10. Boosts mood
11. Reduces risk of falls

How Much Do you Need:

Around 30 minutes of moderate cardiovascular activity is recommended[1] at least 5x per week.

Muscular Conditioning (or strength training)

Is the maximum amount of force that your muscles can exert in a single maximal effort. The three most effective ways to improve your muscular strength and endurance are by using the resistance of your own body weight (such as push-ups, squats, or lunges), free weights (dumbbells), or exercise machines. What method you choose is determined by your goals, availability of equipment, limitations due to previous injuries, and personal preferences.

Benefits of strong muscles:

1. Improves your posture
2. Reduces your risk of injury
3. Makes your everyday activities easier
4. Preserves muscle mass
5. Controls weight
6. Reduces risk of osteoporosis

How Much Do you Need:

It is recommended to perform strength training exercises a minimum of 2x per week[1].

---

1   https://www.participaction.com/en-ca/benefits-and-guidelines/adults-18-to-64

Flexibility (or stretching)

Is the range of motion around each of your individual joints. Flexibility is improved by stretching, which means to exert a slight amount of tension on the joints and hold it there for about 10 seconds to three minutes.

Benefits:

Flexibility helps decrease your risk of injury and muscle soreness after a workout, helps prevent lower back pain, improves physical performance, and improves your circulation.

How Much Do you Need:

Stretching can be performed everyday as long as you're not overdoing it. If you're new to stretching, you can start with just five minutes per day or 15 minutes 3x per week.

The bottom line: Good fitness involves strength and efficiency in all three areas, and overworking any one while neglecting the others can lead to problems. To maximize fat loss your goal is to burn more calories than you consume, so begin by increasing the amount of activity you're currently performing.

Reflect

Why was it important for the Proverbs 31 woman to be strong?

_____

_____

_____

_____

_____

Why is it important for you to be strong?

_____

_____

_____

_____

_____

Of the three components of fitness, which would you benefit from the most?

_____

_____

_____

_____

_____

Pray

Dear Lord, I thank You for making me so perfectly. I'm in awe of Your perfect design. My heart pumps blood to my entire body, my strong muscles give me the ability to do work, and the flexibility at my joints keeps me supple and limber. Forgive me for not treating my body as the true wonder that it is. Let me never take any of my body systems for granted. As I go through this study this month, let me 'rise up' and glorify You in my body. Let me move my body and learn to celebrate it as the gift that it truly is. And mostly, give me the desire to begin to exercise daily. In Your Name I pray!

My Prayer

_____
_____
_____
_____
_____
_____
_____
_____
_____
_____
_____
_____
_____
_____
_____
_____
_____
_____

Additional Scriptures

"Do you not know that your body is a temple of the Holy Spirit who is in you, whom you have received from God? You are not your own." (1 Corinthians 6:19 NIV)

"For physical training is of some value, but godliness has value for all things, holding promise for both the present life and the life to come." (1 Timothy 4:8 NIV)

Day 3:

Rise Up and say 'Yes'

Scripture Reflection

> *"When Jesus saw him lying there and learned that he had been in this condition for a long time, he asked him, "Do you want to get well?"* (John 5:6 NKJV)

Devotion

Jesus asked the infirmed man, *"Do you want to get well?"*

Seems like an obvious question, right?

Maybe on the surface, but Jesus knows that not everyone who says they want to be well really means it.

God knows that, as painful as our current situations are, we choose comfort, complacency, and familiarity over the unknown. Change requires work, and are we truly ready to do what it takes?

If you're really honest with yourself, how would you answer the question, *"Do you want to get well?"*

"I really do, but..."

"I don't want to get too obsessive about this fitness thing."

"I really do, but I'm not sure if I can maintain it"

"I only have so much time in the day."

"I have to take my pills, so I have to eat ...."

"I have an injury, so I can't really push myself that hard."

Jesus' question to the man at the pool (and to us) challenges us to truly explore our desires, our commitment, our motives, and our trust in Him. Do you want to be made well? As you go through this challenge, be honest in your answer to this question. Can you answer with a resounding, "YES!"? If not, ask God to give you the grace, strength, and desire to let go of your fears and doubts, and to truly desire His best for you. As you begin to release your fears to God, you will be more inspired and encouraged to move your body more and get healthier each day.

Reflect

Why did Jesus ask the man if he wanted to get well? Wouldn't Jesus know that he 'obviously' would want to?

_____

_____

_____

_____

_____

_____

Has Jesus 'questioned' you about your intention and commitment to exercise or getting healthier? Has your response been a "yes, but?" What is your 'but'?

_____
_____
_____
_____
_____

What will it take to commit to a resounding 'yes' today?

_____
_____
_____
_____
_____

Pray

Dear Lord, I thank You for this challenge. I want to get well, Lord. Come in and remove all the doubts and fears so I can answer with a loud and convincing, YES! It is in You that I live, move, and have my being. So as I embark on this challenge, I commit this journey to You. In Your awesome Name I thank You and praise You, Lord! Amen.

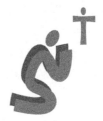

My Prayer

_____
_____
_____
_____
_____
_____
_____
_____
_____
_____

Additional Study Scriptures

*"But let your 'Yes' be 'Yes,' and your 'No,' 'No.' For whatever
is more than these is from the evil one."*
(Matthew 5:37 KJV)

*"But when you ask, you must believe and not doubt, because
the one who doubts is like a wave of the sea, blown and
tossed by the wind. That person should not expect to receive
anything from the Lord. Such a person is double-minded and
unstable in all they do."*
(James 1:6–8 NIV)

*"He saith unto him the third time, Simon, son of Jonas, lovest
thou me? Peter was grieved because he said unto him the
third time, Lovest thou me? And he said unto him, Lord, thou
knowest all things; thou knowest that I love thee. Jesus saith
unto him, Feed my sheep."*
(John 21:17 KJV)

Day 4:

Rise Up and Go North

Scripture Reflection

> *"You have circled this mountain long enough.*
> *Now turn north."*
> (Deut 2:3 NASB)

Devotion

How long have you been wanting to get in better shape? It's probably been a long time, but for one reason or another you keep putting it off. This book and challenge are designed to move you into action by helping you to align with God's Word. It's time to take action.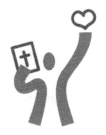

Similarly to Jesus telling the infirm man at Bethesda to rise up, God also delivered a message to Moses. While wandering in the desert, God spoke to Moses and said, *"Listen up, you've been in this place long enough—go north."*

You may be feeling stuck like the infirm man at the pool, waiting for a miracle, or you may be feeling like the Israelites on a journey for 40 years, desperately hoping for the Promised

Land. But from your vantage point, it seems like it may never happen for you.

Wherever you find yourself, know that today is a new day and it's time for a change. It's time to do a new thing. It's time to stop circling the same mountain, and 'go north'—upward and onward towards a healthier life.

The Israelites were wandering in the desert; the man was lying at a pool. Two extremes, yet their struggle was similar— they were both stuck in a cycle.

Jesus' question to him exposed just how stuck he was in his pattern. Jesus was speaking to the condition of the man's heart when He asked him if he wanted to get well. Regardless of whether you've been stuck because you have a physical infirmity, whether you fell out of the habit and find it hard to restart, or because you're just not motivated, it's time to go north.

Yes, you may backslide sometimes, but it's all good. God is not asking for perfection. He's looking for progress.

Yes, the journey will be difficult and your flesh may be kicking and screaming. But God promises that He will be with you in the midst of it and He will give you the strength to bear up under it.

Are you ready to go north?

Reflect

How is the Lord leading you to 'go north'?

What has gotten in the way as you've tried to move forward in the past?

How do you believe this time will be different?

Pray

Lord, I'm so tired of circling the same mountains in my life. I'm so tired of my own disobedience and rebelliousness, yet I'm not sure I know how to live any other way. I've been doing it my way for so long that I don't even recognize it, Lord. Open my eyes so I can see a new direction. I will look up and fix my eyes on You. I surrender my habits, my proclivities, my will, and my ways to You, Lord. I'm ready to make exercise part of my daily lifestyle. In Your Name I pray. Amen.

My Prayer

_____
_____
_____
_____
_____
_____
_____
_____
_____
_____

Additional Study Scriptures

"And call on me in the day of trouble; I will deliver you, and you will honor me."
(Psalm 50:15 NIV)

"Let your eyes look straight ahead; fix your gaze directly before you. Give careful thought to the paths for your feet and be steadfast in all your ways. Do not turn to the right or the left; keep your foot from evil."
(Proverbs 4:25–27 NIV)

"See, I am doing a new thing! Now it springs up; do you not perceive it? I am making a way in the wilderness and streams in the wasteland."
(Isaiah 43:19 NIV)

Day 5:

Rise Up and Manage Your Expectations

Scripture Reflection

> *"Are You the Expected One, or shall we look for someone else?"* (Matthew 11:3 NASB)

Devotion

What's your expectation while you're in this challenge? Do you have high expectations that you will suddenly transform your body into a daily workout machine? Or maybe you have very low expectations and think that you're not going to be successful and will probably lose steam after a few days.

There's an expression that says, *'You get what you expect.'* Put another way, your success will be determined by your level of expectation.

But what if you've traditionally had low expectations? Or unrealistic expectations?

The secret to meeting your expectations is to spend time with God and let Him set the expectation based on His best for you. Line up your expectations with scripture from the Bible instead of what you think will or will not happen.

In the Bible, John the Baptist also had unrealistic expectations about what Jesus would be like. He preached about Jesus' kingdom coming with power and justice. But instead, Jesus preached about love and acts of mercy. John even sent messengers to ask Jesus, "Are you the Expected One, or shall we look for someone else?" (Matthew 11:3)

Jesus' response was to challenge John the Baptist's expectations and encourage him to base it on the Word of God instead of what he thought Jesus would be like. "And blessed is he who does not take offense at Me." (Matthew 11:6)

Like John, are you holding on to expectations about what you think this journey should be like? Or maybe you have certain beliefs about how God should be working in your life. Maybe you want Him to give you more motivation, or remove some things from your life so you can have more time.

And what about the man at the pool? He had an expectation that someone would help him into the pool, and that unfulfilled expectation left him in a state of helplessness and despair. This can easily set in when we hold on to our expectations without letting the Holy Spirit lead us.

Remember, we can't see the entire picture. And we most certainly will never be able to comprehend the mind of God. We do know that His ways are higher than our ways (Isaiah 55:8), and that's why we must let go of our expectations and trust Him for our outcome.

Yes, it's good to have dreams, goals, visions, and expectations, but let go of how you think you will get there. Don't be so attached to the outcome or how the journey should look. Hold loosely to the picture. We don't know how God will show up, but you can be sure that He always will.

Reflect

John the Baptist clearly recognized Jesus as the Messiah, but his expectations about what Jesus should do were misguided. Do you have expectations about how and what the Lord should and should not do to deliver you from your strongholds?

_____

_____

_____

_____

_____

What beliefs do you have about how the Lord should be working in your life? Surrender them to Him today and trust that His ways are best.

_____

_____

_____

_____

_____

Are there some expectations that you need to possibly grieve and let go of? Maybe you thought you would have achieved your goal by now. Or by 40, 50, or 60 you would have done 'X'. What-ever those unfulfilled expectations are, give them to God by ac-cepting, acknowledging, and standing in a new possibility.

_____
_____
_____
_____
_____

Pray

Father God, I surrender my will and my ways to You. Your thoughts are higher than my thoughts and Your ways are higher than my ways. Keep me mindful of that when I forget. I love You, Lord, and give you all my expectations and desires. Continue to line up my expectations with Yours and then help me to develop habits that match those expectations. I surrender it all to You. Amen!

My Prayer

_____
_____
_____
_____
_____
_____
_____
_____
_____
_____
_____
_____

Additional Study Scriptures

"For my thoughts are not your thoughts,
neither are your ways my ways,"
(Isaiah 55:8 NIV)

"Yes, my soul, find rest in God;
my hope comes from him."
(Psalm 62:5 NIV)

Day 6:

Seeing Exercise From a Different Perspective

Scripture Reflection

"Do not conform to the pattern of this world, but be transformed by the renewing of your mind. Then you will be able to test and approve what God's will is—his good, pleasing and perfect will." (Romans 12:2 NIV)

Devotion

Close cousins to your attitude, which we talked about yesterday, is your perspective. They both play very important roles in determining the success and failure of your ability to adhere to an exercise routine, or any other goal in life for that matter.

If you perceive exercise as a form of punishment, you will continue to avoid it.

If you've latched on to old beliefs or messages like, "No pain, no gain", you will continue to avoid it.

If you believe you have to devote hours a day to make it worth your while, you will continue to procrastinate until you can find the time.

And if you perceive that exercise is hard, confusing, overwhelming, embarrassing, and just unpleasant—once again, it will be difficult to make it a consistent part of your routine.

That's why it's important to pay attention to your perception of exercise and learn new skills, mindsets, and habits to change your perspective.

Romans 12:2 reminds us not to think as the world thinks. Instead, we are to put everything through the lens of God. Ask yourself, "Is this in line with God's will for me?" If it isn't (and why wouldn't it be), then it's time to reframe exercise. Below is how you can begin to change your perspective about exercise.

See Exercise as a Form of Worship to God

Many of us think of exercise as a painful, boring, time-consuming nuisance. Have you ever thought about what God thinks about exercise? I don't mean the sweating, hardcore bodies working out at a gym. I'm talking about how He feels about you spending time with Him, worshiping Him with your body. Begin to change your mind and attitude about exercise by seeing it from His perspective.

Start Slow and Easy

Many of us get overly ambitious when we decide to start. We're sore for many days after; we may have even injured something and now have a negative association with exercise. Start with one push up against the wall if that's all you want to do. The important thing is to just start somewhere and gradually build up.

Make it Fit with Your Personality

Are you an introvert? Try swimming laps in a pool. Social but-terfly? Try a Zumba or aqua-fit class. Competitive? Register and begin training for a race. Love the outdoors? Hiking is a great form of exercise. If you're easily bored, then continue to vary your routine. Create a list of 5-10 different things you like and change them frequently. Many of us have been forced to believe that exercise should look and feel a certain way in order to be effective. This is simply not true. Find what works for you and do it.

Focus on Daily Progress

Some days you can hardly wait to exercise, and some days the thought of it will make you want to jump back into bed. It's all good. As long as you do something each day, you will contin-ue to make progress. Listen to your body. Since it knows that exercise is good for you, it will rarely tell you not to do it. Your mind, on the other hand ... that, you will have to ignore a lot of the time.

Don't Make It Optional

Unfortunately, many of us see exercise as a luxury for those blessed with the gift of time or with the luxury of going to the gym or reserved for people with willpower or discipline. It's these beliefs that keep us from making it a habit. Exercise should be part of our daily routine, as natural as brushing your teeth and taking a shower each day. When you can begin to see it as part of your daily routine, then you will make time for it and begin to look for ways to incorporate it into your daily schedule.

These shifts will go a long way in helping you to change your perspective on exercise.

Reflect

What is your belief about how long you need to exercise in order to see results? Write out a healthy perspective about this belief such as 'Every little bit helps'.

_____

_____

_____

_____

_____

_____

Reread Romans 12:2. How will you renew your mind so that you can begin to think differently about exercise?

_____

_____

_____

_____

_____

_____

Journal what your new healthy perspective about exercise will look like once you've renewed your mind and released all the limiting beliefs.

_____

_____

_____

_____

_____

_____

Pray

Dear Lord, forgive me for neglecting my body by not moving it and giving it the exercise that it needs. When I don't 'feel' like exercising, remind me to move past my feelings. When I don't have the time, remind me to prioritize what's important. And when I feel discouraged and it feels too hard, give me strength, Lord. Help me 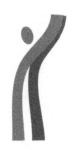 to see exercise as a daily form of worship to You. Let me celebrate you every time I move my body. Let me use that time to pray for others, to fix my mind on You, and to be thankful for how wonderfully You created my body. In Jesus' Name, amen.

My Prayer

_____

_____

_____

_____

_____

_____

_____

_____

_____

_____

Additional Study Scriptures

"Now, therefore, make a confession to the LORD, the God of your fathers, and do His will. Separate yourselves from the people of the land and from your foreign wives."
(Ezra 10:11 NIV)

"No discipline seems pleasant at the time, but painful. Later on, however, it produces a harvest of righteousness and peace for those who have been trained by it."
(Hebrews 12:11 NIV)

Day 7:

Week 1 Reflections

Scripture Reference

"Give thanks in all circumstances;
for this is the will of God in Christ Jesus for you."
(1 Thessalonians 5:18 ESV)

1. Recap

Review the first week of devotions and journal any new insights that you've learned. What are you discovering about yourself as it relates to exercise and staying active?

_____

_____

_____

_____

_____

2. Reflect

Journal what the Holy Spirit is showing you so far. How will this new habit help you align with your word for the year?

_____

_____

---

3. Pray

Commit your week to the Lord. Rest in Him and allow Him to give you the spirit of self-control and discipline.

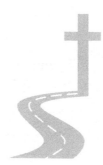

Day 8:
Designing Your Exercise Program - Your 21-Day Challenge

Scripture Reflection

> *"Suppose one of you wants to build a tower. Won't you first sit down and estimate the cost to see if you have enough money to complete it?"* (Luke 14:28 NIV)

Devotion

We use this scripture a lot in my Weight Loss, God's Way membership program. Why? Because we understand the importance of planning and preparation. The same is true for your exercise program. Sure, you can just go outside and start walking, which would be fantastic, but if you have specific goals in mind you will need to tailor your program (weightlossgodsway.com).

If you currently do not have an exercise program, follow these steps to help you get started. As we already discussed in the Exercise 101 lesson, your program should incorporate an aerobic (cardio-vascular) component, a strengthening (muscle conditioning) component, and a stretching (flexibility) component.

Choose from one of the following categories:

Beginner – If you currently do very little to no exercise, your challenge is to simply do something every day. It does not matter what you do, but do something each day. It could be as simple to some light stretching, to walking, to one of the workouts.

Intermediate – If you currently exercise but you're not consistent, you're going to commit to exercising for a minimum of 15 minutes per day, every day. This can include walking, muscle conditioning, or even stretching. The focus is on consistency.

Advanced – If you exercise consistently but you're not seeing results, you're going to focus on either adding muscular conditioning (weight training) to your workouts or do something different than you're accustomed to doing. If you're a more advanced exerciser, follow the guidelines below:

Then every day, for the next twenty-one days, commit to honoring your commitment each day. To help you stay motivated and focused, here are a few additional exercise guidelines.

Balance the intensity of your workouts

I encourage clients to be focused and intense when they are exercising. However, not all of your workouts should be at the same intensity. I usually encourage one intense day, one moderate day, and one lighter day per week when doing both aerobic exercise and muscle conditioning. When all your workouts are the same high intensity, your body can get overstressed and you can actually start to experience negative effects.

Think of your weekly routine if you have one. Are some workouts more challenging than others? If not, how can you change it up to vary the intensity?

Balance your work/rest ratio

Rest is just as important as exercising. Your body needs to rest both during your workouts and also on the days when you are not exercising.

Rest periods during your workouts are important during weight training or muscular conditioning exercises when you want to shape and tone your muscles. Studies have found that both testosterone and the growth hormone are produced in greater levels when you rest for short to moderate periods; 60 to 90 seconds between sets seems to be the agreed upon rest time in the fitness world.

Rest periods are also important between your workout days. One of the most common questions I get asked is, "Is it okay to work out every day?"

Here is my usual response:

For cardiovascular fitness it's okay to exercise every day, as long as you balance your workout by alternating between intense days and light days.

For muscle toning and strengthening, I recommend 48 hours between muscle groups. That means if you train your legs on Monday, then your next leg workout would be on Wednesday or later.

Why rest days?

It's actually on your rest days that your muscles get stronger. On your rest days the muscles you trained get repaired and healed. If you have not had adequate rest, your body cannot regenerate itself. Without adequate rest you run the risk of injury, you may not get the results you're looking for, and you may even see a decrease in your performance.

Balance your upper body and lower body

Do you spend as much time on your upper body as you do on your lower body? Men tend to spend more time on their upper body, especially the bench press, while women tend to spend too much time on their lower body, especially the inner and outer thigh machines. Resist the urge to focus on one or the other.

If your current routine is only walking, think about adding some hand weights or upper body exercises to your routine.

Reflect

What habits, mindsets, or systems will you need to put in place for you to be successful over the next 21 days?

_____

_____

_____

_____

_____

What are some of the benefits of exercise that you are looking forward to experiencing?

_____

_____

_____

_____

_____

What will you do if you miss a day? Write out a contingency plan.

_____

_____

_____

_____

_____

Pray

Lord, I thank You for this 21-day, get-active challenge. Help me to step out of my comfort zone and not be afraid to push myself within healthy limits. I know that challenges change me, but I want these changes to last more than 21 days. I want these changes to be for the rest of my life. So remind me, Lord, 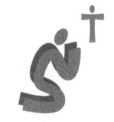 that this is the start of a new life-long habit that will bring You glory. Strengthen me when I'm feeling unmotivated, and at the end of this challenge I want to hear you say, "Well done, good and faithful servant".

My Prayer

_____

_____

_____

_____

_____

_____

_____

_____

_____

_____

_____

_____

_____

_____

Day 9:

Feelings Aren't Facts

Scripture Reflection

"A person without self-control is like a house with its doors and windows knocked out." (Proverbs 25:28 MSG)

Devotion

Last week, you said 'yes' to God, but today is another day. Are you still experiencing the warm, fuzzy feelings that you had when you made that declaration, or are they already starting to fade? Has life started to get in the way.

How do you continue to say "yes" to God each and every day?

- You say 'yes' to God every time you say no to your flesh.

- You say 'yes' to God every time you choose faith over your fears.

- You say 'yes' to God when you refuse to let life's other priorities try to squeeze out your exercise time.

- You say 'yes' to God when you put yourself first and realize that you're not being selfish. You're actually honoring God.

- You say 'yes' to God every time you obey His Word.

- You say 'yes' to God when you take action despite what you're feeling.

Remember, feelings aren't facts. In fact, they are very fickle—they change from moment to moment, and are easily influenced by our flesh.

The scripture above makes the analogy between lack of self-control and a house without windows and doors. It acknowledges that lack of self-control (and a house without walls) leaves you vulnerable to attacks and provides no safety or protection. When we lack self-control by giving in to our feelings we also leave ourselves vulnerable to attacks from the enemy, from the lure of worldly influences, and from our thoughts and beliefs.

Fast forward to the end of the story of the infirm man at the pool in Bethesda and you'll discover that the man at the pool showed faith when He obeyed Jesus' command. God's Spirit stirred up something in him that allowed him to rise up and walk. That same spirit lives in you, and will also stir you to take action regardless of what you're feeling.

Choose to live by the Spirit of God that lives in you and refuse to be led by your feelings. They're fickle, and will often talk you out of doing what you know you should do.

Pay attention to when your feelings are trying to run the show. It often sounds like this:

I 'should' exercise

I 'should not' take time for myself

I 'need' a break

When the spirit of God quickens you, you won't be feeling guilty and you won't be "should-ing" yourself. You will rise up and take action.

You've got this, with the Lord as your strength.

Reflect

How are you constantly 'should-ing' yourself (or saying 'need to', 'have to', and 'want to'), and how does this language keep you from taking action?

_____
_____
_____
_____
_____

Where/how do you lack self-control when it comes to staying active and exercising?

_____
_____
_____
_____
_____

If you miss a day, how will you keep from experiencing feelings of guilt?

_____

_____

_____

_____

_____

Pray

Lord, I say 'Yes" to You. I say 'yes' to Your will and Your ways. I say 'yes' to Your Spirit that dwells in me and compels me to live in faith and not fear as I exercise today. I thank You for the ability to move my body and give You glory. I choose to be led by Your Spirit instead of by my feelings. Keep reminding me of how fickle my feelings are. They are not the final word. In Your precious Name I pray! Amen.

My Prayer

_____

_____

_____

_____

_____

_____

_____

_____

Additional Scriptures

"Even if we feel guilty, God is greater than our feelings, and he knows everything."
(1 John 3:20 NLT)

"The heart is deceitful above all things and beyond cure. Who can understand it?"
(Jeremiah 17:9 NIV)

"Whoever trusts in his own mind is a fool, but he who walks in wisdom will be delivered."
(Proverbs 28:6 ESV)

Day 10:

Rise Up and Take Baby Steps

Scripture Reflection

"Little by little I will drive them out before you until you have increased enough to take possession of the land."
(Exodus 23:30 NIV)

Devotion

Your success in this challenge and in maintaining a consistent fitness routine is based on developing small, daily, consistent habits.

Resist the urge to feel like to you have to make massive transformations in your life. And you don't need to start by working out for hours a day. Start where you're at and gradually increase. What are some small things you can do each day to include more movement in your life?

Unfortunately, shows like *The Biggest Loser* would have us believe that we need to put in hours of training a day, but that's not reality.

As the Israelites marched out of Egypt, through the Red Sea and into the wilderness, God promised He would be with them through the entire journey. He also promised that He would help them have victory over all of their enemies, and was very specific on how He would help them. God says, "I will drive them out little by little until you have increased enough to take possession of the land." (Exodus 23:30)

Why would an all-powerful God take His time to act? God understands that to be victorious certain skills must be developed, such as persistence, patience, strategy, and submission. These qualities are not developed overnight. God wants us to get the lessons as well as blessings.

You will be victorious making fitness become a lifestyle as you learn to take it step-by-step.

Reflect

Most of us are not thrilled about the idea of baby steps. We would rather change quickly and significantly. What are some problems with change that happens quickly and drastically?

_____

_____

_____

_____

_____

_____

_____

God cared for the Israelites and wanted them to grow little by little so that they could increase. How can God work in your life more effectively when you take steps 'little by little'?

_____
_____
_____
_____
_____
_____

What little steps have you already been taking? Give God thanks for them all.

_____
_____
_____
_____
_____
_____

Pray

Dear Lord, If I'm being totally honest, even though it has taken me years to develop some of my bad habits, I don't like the idea of baby steps. I've wasted so much time already. I want to accelerate my results. But I know that fast won't last. I know that I will burn out quickly and that I will miss great lessons that You're trying to teach me. Teach me how to be grateful with the progress I'm making, even though it's slower than I would like. Teach me to let go of wanting results quickly and give me Your peace about this process no matter how long it takes. In Your Name I pray. Amen!

My Prayer

_____
_____
_____
_____
_____
_____
_____
_____
_____
_____
_____
_____
_____
_____
_____

Additional Study Scriptures

"Do not despise these small beginnings, for the Lord rejoices to see the work begin, to see the plumb line in Zerubbabel's hand." (Zechariah 4:10 NLT)

"So He said, 'Truly I say to you that this poor widow has put in more than all; for all these out of their abundance have put in offerings for God, but she out of her poverty put in all the livelihood that she had.'" (Luke 21:3-4 NKJV)

Day 11:

Rise Up and Make Time

Scripture Reflection

> *"... making the most of your time,*
> *because the days are evil."*
> (Ephesians 5:16 NASB)

Devotion

One of the biggest reasons people give for not exercising is a lack of time.

So today let's bust this 'time myth', because it's robbing you of your health.

Here's the thing—we all have the same exact amount of time each and every day. No one gets one minute more or less. So how is it that some people are able to manage their time effectively and efficiently, while some of us are constantly feeling like we're always chasing our tails?

Truth is, if time is your biggest enemy, you don't have a time problem. You have a priority problem.

We struggle with time because ...

- Our priorities are out of order

- We base our time on what we think we should be doing or what feels urgent instead of letting God manage our time

- We've filled our lives with too many things that God never called us to do in the first place

Once you get a true revelation of what you were put on this earth to do and who you are here to serve, then you will no longer have a time issue. You will learn to work your priorities and let go of the rest. Time will only become an issue when you put your agenda ahead of God's.

God has given us just enough time to do what He's called us to—to live out our assignment. That's our priority. We waste time because we veer off in other directions, because we give in to peer pressure, we want to please others, we want to satisfy our flesh, or we listen to the lies of the enemy telling us to focus on something other than what God has called us to. Even though it may feel productive but God did not call you to do it, you will feel like you've wasted your time.

It's in spending time with God that we learn how to focus on our priorities. We find our purpose and our priorities in Him. When you make time for God, you will have the time to do what He has called you to do and you will learn to let go of the rest.

May we be a people who understand our priorities, make time for God, and make time to maintain our health. May we be children who make the most of our days. How will you make time to exercise today?

Reflect

Think about how you prioritize your time. How can you change your priorities to make time for exercise?

_____
_____
_____
_____
_____
_____

What robs you of your time? Pray about it and develop a plan to eliminate it from your life.

_____
_____
_____
_____
_____
_____

How can you make the most of your time as Ephesians 5:16 tells us?

_____
_____
_____
_____
_____
_____

Pray

Dear Lord God, I'm thankful for this time with You right now! This lesson is hard to hear, Father, and I'm grateful for the conviction I feel. I confess and repent of trying to be the general manager of the time You've given me, and today I surrender my agenda to You! Managing my time is an inside-out job that I need You in charge of, Lord. I'm asking Your Holy Spirit to reorganize my mind and re-center my heart on You. Search me and show me the ways that my priorities are mixed up, clarify for me whatever may have first place in my heart, and convict me to surrender that which doesn't belong in that precious spot. Help me make time in my day to exercise and strengthen my temple. I want to thank You, Father, for the blessing of the wonderful time I get to spend here on earth, with the people that I love and in communion with You. Whatever I truly desire I will naturally make time for. My intention is to use each moment of the time given to me for Your glory! Amen.

My Prayer

_____

_____

_____

_____

_____

_____

_____

_____

_____

_____

Additional Study Scriptures

"Walk in wisdom toward outsiders, making the best use of the time." (Colossians 4:5 ESV)

"I glorified you on earth, having accomplished the work that you gave me to do." (John 17:4 ESV)

Day 12:
Rise Up and Keep Walking Forward

Scripture Reflection

> *"Then Jesus said to him, 'Get up! Pick up your mat and walk.'"* (John 5:8 KJV)

Devotion

Why did Jesus tell the man at the pool to take up his bed (mat)? The miracle was powerful in itself, don't you think? Someone paralyzed for 38 years, now had the ability to get up and walk!

But Jesus wanted more from him. Not only did he want the man to move forward in his life, but He did not want him returning to what was familiar. He did not want Him to go back to his mat. It's symbolic that he was now carrying the very thing that had carried him for so many years. How powerful is that? He was now in charge of his future. The memory of 38 years on a mat did not have to dictate how he would live the rest of his life.

It is so easy to return to the familiar when you experience a setback. The comfort and security of your mat (past) can feel very safe, despite how much it keeps you bound.

God is calling us to forget our former ways and move forward in the new direction that He is calling us. No looking back, no returning to your old, familiar mat—don't even remember the pool. Staying stuck in the past will never allow you to move into your future. Forward movement only!

"Remember not the former things, nor consider the things of old. Behold, I am doing a new thing; now it springs forth, do you not perceive it? I will make a way in the wilderness and rivers in the desert." (Isaiah 43:18–19 ESV)

If you keep slipping back into old, familiar habits of not exercising, stop and pay attention to what you're telling yourself. Are you telling yourself that it's too hard? You'll do it tomorrow? You're too tired? The more you continue feeding these stories to yourself, the more you will remain stuck on your mat. Rise up today, take up your bed, and walk!

Reflect

In regard to your fitness and activity level, what unproductive situations or scenarios do you keep returning to?

_____

_____

_____

_____

_____

_____

_____

_____

_____

How is God calling you to 'rise up' and look at your health differently?

_____

_____

_____

_____

_____

_____

Jesus challenged the man to do the impossible (through the lens of our human eyes). What is He calling you to do on this health journey that seems impossible? Will you trust Him?

_____

_____

_____

_____

_____

_____

Pray

Dear Lord, I'm not looking back. I'm committed to finishing this challenge, and am committed to remaining active and healthy for as long as it is Your will. I'm committing to my health and I'm committed to You. I've taken up my mat and I recognize that it has served its purpose. I'm not going back, and I declare that there will always be forward movement. I am a new creation in You! Amen.

My Prayer

_____
_____
_____
_____
_____
_____
_____
_____
_____
_____
_____
_____
_____
_____
_____

Additional Study Scriptures

*"Therefore, if anyone is in Christ, the new creation has come:
The old has gone, the new is here!"* (2 Cor 5:17 NIV)

*"'Aeneas,' Peter said to him, 'Jesus Christ heals you.
Get up and roll up your mat.' Immediately Aeneas got up."*
(Acts 9:34 NIV)

Day 13:

Rise Up and Find Motivation in God

Scripture Reflection

> *"For in him we live and move and have our being."*
> (Acts 17:28 NIV)

Devotion

Studies show that people who exercise because they 'should' or because they 'need to' lose weight, are not able to maintain their motivation. Feelings of 'should,' 'need to,' and 'have to' only produce feelings of guilt, which are not good motivators to do anything.

If you truly want to develop a fitness program that will become a lifestyle, instead of another program that you end up quitting, do the following:

a. Focus on renewing your mind with the Word of God instead of trying to 'make' yourself exercise.

Romans 12:2– The Word says that we are transformed by renewing our mind, meaning that change comes from the inside out. Change the way you think first in order to see external changes. Speak the Word of God over your health, your habits, and your mind. Confront all of your challenges, excuses, and fears with the Word of God. It is the only thing able to cut through all of the resistance you face.

b. Focus on long-term success for your body, soul (emotions and will), and spirit instead of on quick fixes.

Proverbs 28:19-20 reminds us that quick fixes and shortcuts will never last. Find motivation by thinking about a life-long fitness habit that becomes part of your daily life. Take yourself through a series of questions before jumping in. Ask yourself, "Is this something that I can maintain?" and/or "How will God be glorified by my actions?" "What is my motivation for taking on this program?" "How is this part of a bigger picture?"

c. Focus on submitting this journey to God and pray for the motivation, discipline, and strength to make the time to exercise each day.

It's funny how many people never considered inviting God into their workouts, or their weight loss journey. We reserve God for what we consider spiritual things and think He's not interested in our day to day activities. Where did that belief ever come from? We miss out on so much when we relegate God to only certain areas of our lives. Recognize that God cares about everything that we care about, so don't be afraid to invite Him in. He will strengthen you for the journey.

You've got this with the Lord as your strength!

Reflect

How have you been trying to get more fit in your own strength in the past? How well has it worked out for you?

_____

_____

_____

_____

_____

Have you ever asked God to give you the discipline to maintain a fitness program? If not, ask Him today.

_____

_____

_____

_____

_____

How can you incorporate all of your being—your body, soul, and spirit—into your fitness program?

_____

_____

_____

_____

_____

Pray

Lord, my desire is to let my motivation come from You, and You alone. After the excitement fades, I want to commit to moving my body each and every day. I truly want to glorify You. Let me see the ability to exercise not as a form of punishment, but as a privilege! I'm so grateful that I get to move every day. Let me never take that for granted. In Jesus' Name, I pray. Amen.

My Prayer

_____

_____

_____

_____

_____

_____

_____

_____

_____

_____

Additional Study Scriptures

"We are destroying sophisticated arguments and every exalted and proud thing that sets itself up against the [true] knowledge of God, and we are taking every thought and purpose captive to the obedience of Christ."
(2 Cor 10:5)

*"For the word of God is alive and active.
Sharper than any double-edged sword, it penetrates even to dividing soul and spirit, joints and marrow; it judges the thoughts and attitudes of the heart."*
(Hebrews 4:12 NIV)

Day 14:

Week 2 Reflections

Scripture Reference

"Give thanks in all circumstances; for this is the will of God in Christ Jesus for you." (1 Thessalonians 5:18 ESV)

1. Recap: This week...

Review the last seven devotions and journal any new insights that you've learned. What are you discovering about yourself as it relates to exercise and staying active?

_____
_____
_____
_____
_____
_____
_____
_____
_____
_____
_____
_____
_____
_____

2. Reflect

Journal what the Holy Spirit is showing you so far. How will this new habit help you align with your word for the year?

_____

_____

_____

_____

_____

_____

_____

_____

_____

3. Pray

Commit your week to the Lord. Rest in Him and allow Him to give you the spirit of self-control and discipline.

_____

_____

_____

_____

_____

_____

_____

_____

_____

Day 15:

Rise Up and Accept God's Discipline

Scripture Reflection

> *"No discipline seems pleasant at the time, but painful. Later on, however, it produces a harvest of righteousness and peace for those who have been trained by it."* (Hebrews 12:11 NIV)

Devotion

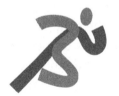

Let's be honest. It takes discipline to exercise.

It takes discipline to wake up early when you don't feel like it. And put on your shoes, break a sweat, and endure the pain of aching muscles.

Some people are naturally more disciplined than others. It could be their natural personality, their upbringing, their ability to forgo gratification, or a deep sense of understanding that short-term discomfort is better than long-term regret.

Regardless of where you fall on the spectrum of discipline, Hebrews 12:11 teaches us an important principle about discipline. In order for us to benefit from God's discipline, we must be "trained" by it. God has a purpose in training us.

This training is necessary for God to strengthen our spiritual muscles. If we try to bypass or forego the pain of training, we will pay for it later by being defeated by temptation and sin. We will continually feel in bondage if we keep satisfying our flesh by enjoying the immediate pleasure instead of 'suffering' through the temporary pain. We can't have both.

This exact principle applies to our physical bodies when it comes to training. *Yeah, but it's still hard,* you might be saying.

So just how do we learn discipline? The key is not in ourselves, but to look upward. Discipline is a gift we receive from the Holy Spirit. It is not something we can muster up in our own strength. Our role as Hebrews 12:11 teaches us is to accept the training.

Exercise will require us to continually train ourselves to bring our flesh and our desires under the control of Christ by the power of His Spirit. Yes, it is not pleasant at the time, but we must continually train ourselves to look beyond the immediate pain. God would never command us to do something and make it too difficult (Deut. 30:11). There is much pleasure for us to experience at the end of the journey if we accept God's training. It's worth it! You're worth it!

Reflect

Change the way you view discipline and see it as a form of training, not punishment. How does this perspective help you to embrace exercise?

_____
_____
_____
_____
_____

How will you continually bring your flesh under submission?

_____
_____
_____
_____
_____

How will disciplining yourself with exercise help you with discipline in other areas of your life? What other areas of your life will benefit?

_____
_____
_____
_____
_____

Pray

Dear Lord, thank You that You love me enough to want to discipline me! Your desire to shape and mold me comes from Your deep Fatherly love and affection for me, which I'm so grateful for. I will admit it doesn't always feel comfortable in the moment—almost never, actually. But I'm growing in my understanding as I get to know You more intimately as my good Father. Today I ask You to please give me a fresh revelation of Your love for me and a picture of how Your will for me will actually lead me to the best possible outcome. Give me the patience to tolerate the momentary discomfort of going without and turn what seems like deprivation into a keen sense of expectation—an expectation of the wonderful blessings You wish to bestow upon me as I grow in maturity in You. Father, please continue to keep my focus on You rather than on me, so that I may see that Your goal is to have Your glory shine in the world. And it does that best when Your kids look like You. I need Your discipline if I'm going to shine for You, Lord! Thank You, sweet Lord Jesus, for the seed of self-control You put in me and the love You show me through teaching me discipline! Amen.

My Prayer

_____

_____

_____

_____

_____

_____

_____

_____

_____

_____

Additional Study Scriptures

"Whoever loves discipline loves knowledge, but he who hates reproof is stupid." (Proverbs 12:1 NIV)

"But I discipline my body and keep it under control, lest after preaching to others I myself should be disqualified." (1 Cor 9:27 ESV)

Day 16:

Rise Up and Exercise as a Form of Worship

Scripture Reflection

"...always giving thanks to God the Father for everything in the name of our Lord Jesus Christ." (Ephesians 5:20 NIV)

Devotion

Many of us think of exercise as a painful, boring, time-consuming nuisance. Or that it's a luxury reserved for people who have extra time on their hands.

Regardless of what side of the fence you fall on, have you ever thought about what God thinks about exercise? I don't mean the sweating, hardcore bodies working out at a gym. I'm talking about how He feels about you spending time to care for your/His temple.

In a previous lesson, we talked about changing your perspective about how you perceive exercise and physical activity. So today, let's focus on one key perspective. EXERCISE AS WORSHIP.

Romans 12:1 tells us to give our bodies to God as a way to worship Him. Giving our bodies to God means to respect your body and take care of it so that you can do the things He has called you to do. This includes a host of things such as healthy eating, adequate sleep, and exercise. Whatever you do can become a form of worship as you acknowledge and glorify God as you do them.

We learn this in Col 3:17, which tells us: "And whatever you do, whether in word or deed, do it all in the name of the Lord Jesus, giving thanks to God the Father through him".

So how can you make exercise a time of worship?

See it as a time to memorize scripture. I had a season in my life when I would recite scripture as I performed my weight sets. First rep, *"I can do all things through Christ who strengthens me."* Second rep, *"My body is the temple of the Holy Spirit who is in me."* Third rep, *"Greater is He who is in me than the one who is in the world."* Fourth rep, *"When I am weak, then I am strong"*, etc. After your workout your body, mind, and spirit will feel renewed.

What else can you do?

- Give thanks for every muscle that you're working— think about how miraculous your body truly is when it's moving.

- Use it as a time of prayer.

- Use it as a time of praise and worship.

- Listen to scripture as you move your body.

- Exercise on behalf of someone else who is unable to.

- See exercise as a ministry.

- See it as a time between you and God when you commit to talking and listening to how he is speaking to you.

It's time to change the way you think about exercise. It's not meant to be a punishment, but rather a reward and privilege.

Reflect

How will seeing exercise as a form of worship challenge and change your approach to exercise?

_____

_____

_____

_____

Reflect on other ways not included on the list above that you can make exercise a time of worship.

_____

_____

_____

_____

Col 3:17 tells us to "*Do everything in the name of the Lord Jesus, giving thanks to God the Father through him.*" Take a moment and do this now.

_____

_____

_____

_____

Pray

Dear Lord, thank You for changing my mind. Thank You for changing my perspective about exercise. As I begin to see it as an opportunity to spend time with You and glorify You, it changes everything! I'm so thankful that I have a body that can move. As I draw closer to You, I feel myself starting to let go of some of the faulty thinking. Exercise is not punishment for not taking care of myself, but rather it's a reward and a gift that I give to my body. I thank You for giving me wisdom and insight, and I look forward to spending time with You then next time I exercise. In Your Name I pray. Amen!

My Prayer

_____

_____

_____

_____

_____

_____

_____

Additional Study Scriptures

"In all thy ways acknowledge him, and he shall direct thy paths." (Proverbs 3:6 KJV)

"And whatever you do, whether in word or deed, do it all in the name of the Lord Jesus, giving thanks to God the Father through him." (Col 3:17 NIV)

Day 17:

Rise Up and Make Exercise a Habit

Scripture Reflection

"Let me hear Your lovingkindness in the morning; for I trust in You. Teach me the way in which I should walk; for to You I lift up my soul." (Psalm 143:8 NASB)

Devotion

By far, one of the biggest challenges people have with exercise is consistency. Sure, you can do it once or twice or even for a month when you're super-motivated, but as soon as you hit a bump in the road it's often one of the first things to go.

So for the next three days, you will learn how to make exercise a habit by understanding the psychology behind how habits are formed.

Habits are thinking patterns, rituals, and behaviors that are performed automatically and subconsciously. Meaning that we do them without thinking.

When you think about it, most of the things we take for granted each day are habits. Such as walking, talking, brushing your teeth, or getting dressed each day or taking a shower.

Habits are difficult to break, which is great when they are good ones like eating healthy and exercising. But not so good when we have habits such as smoking, excessive TV watching, or eating unnutritious foods.

So just how do you change them?

To change habits, there are three aspects to consider:

- Cues—what triggers you to start the behavior

- Routine—the behavior itself; in this case it's exercise

- Reward—what leads you to repeat the behavior

These three elements are known as the 'habit loop'. It's the ongoing interplay of these three things that maintain habits.

Today, let's look at the first essential element for developing a habit—the cue.

The cue is what will trigger your brain to initiate the behavior.

- Your alarm clock going off in the morning is a cue that it's time to wake up.

- Your phone buzzing is cueing you that you have a text message.

In the Bible, we learn that David loved to seek the Lord early in the morning, and Daniel got down on his knees three times a day and prayed and gave thanks before his God (Daniel 6:10 NIV).

They had specific cues that would trigger them to pray. David's cue was the morning time; Daniel's cue was at specific times during the day, and Jesus' cue was whenever he needed to seek the Lord. To learn from these great men, follow their examples and begin to establish a cue to trigger you to make time to exercise.

Cues can include a specific location, time of day, preceding action, an emotional state, or even other people.

- The alarm clock going off in the morning

- The end of the work day

- Attend a scheduled class at the gym

- Take the dog for a walk at the same time each day

- Pack your gym bag and leave it in front of the door

- Leave a bottle of water and your sneakers next to your bed

- Looking at your running shoes in the car

The key is to make it super simple so that you don't have to think about it, and try to do it at the same time every day.

Reflect

Why does the Bible encourage us to seek God early in the morning?

_____
_____
_____
_____
_____

What are some other cues that trigger you to practice specific
healthy habits? List the cue and the habit.

_____
_____
_____
_____
_____

What are some unhealthy cues that you currently have, and how
will you eliminate them?

_____
_____
_____
_____
_____

Pray

Heavenly Father, I thank You that You help me to develop healthy
habits. Help me to pay attention to my body's cues so that I can

do what's best for my health. Let exercise become as simple and natural for me as breathing. I'm tired of always talking my-self out of it. I just want to do it without all the procrastination and excuse-making. I'm looking forward to getting to the place where it's effortless! In Jesus' Name I pray. Amen.

My Prayer

_____
_____
_____
_____
_____
_____
_____
_____
_____
_____

Additional Study Scriptures

"Now when Daniel learned that the decree had been published, he went home to his upstairs room where the windows opened toward Jerusalem.
Three times a day he got down on his knees and prayed, giving thanks to his God, just as he had done before."
(Daniel 6:10 NIV)

"Early will I seek thee." (Psalm 63:1 KJV)

Day 18:

Rise Up and Establish a Routine

Scripture Reflection

"Put into practice what you learned from me, what you heard and saw and realized. Do that, and God, who makes everything work together, will work you into his most excellent harmonies." (Philippians 4:9)

Devotion

Yesterday, you learned about 'the habit loop'.

- The cues—what triggers you to start the behavior

- The routine—the behavior you want to change

- The reward—what leads you to repeat the behavior.

Today, we'll look at the second part of the habit loop: the routine. The routine is an action or behavior. They can be mental, such as a repeated pattern of thinking, or they can be physical, such as always eating popcorn at the movie theatre for instance. This is what really makes a habit, a habit.

Routines provide structure and consistency for your days and your entire life. They are helpful because they save us a lot of time and effort. When we get into our cars, we don't have to think about how to drive because it's part of our daily routine. The same goes for brushing our teeth and turning off a light switch when leaving a room. These routines are learned once they are repeated over and over again. It's the consistent repetition that establishes routines.

Paul tells the Philippians to:

"Put into practice what you learned from me, what you heard and saw and realized. Do that, and God, who makes everything work together, will work you into his most excellent harmonies." (Philippians 4:9)

As you learned yesterday, routines are developed by strong cues (setting an alarm) and a strong reward (which you'll learn about tomorrow).

To learn how to create habits and develop a consistent routine, take the following points into consideration:

- You can never really get rid of habits, but you can develop new habits or routines to replace the old ones.

- Some habits will take longer than others to develop. It might only take 21 days to develop the habit of drinking water consistently, but it might take years to change your habits around sugar or other trigger foods. Understand that each habit is different.

- Negative reinforcements such as punishment are not usually good motivators. In the case of exercise, you can't force yourself to do it, you can't guilt yourself into exercise, and you can't will yourself to do it. The more you try to do it this way, the more you will end up resenting it.

- Give yourself lots of grace and start slowly.

- Give yourself lots of praise for every small thing you do.

- Choose activities that you enjoy. Again, don't try to force yourself to do something because you think it's the right thing for your body. As you go through these exercises, choose the routines that you love and don't do the ones you hate. If you enjoy competition, find something that will challenge you. If you love being out in nature, go for a walk or jog.

- Creating new habits is a 'long game', rather than a short-term goal. The short-term goals are not usually big enough motivators to keep you going over time. See it as a way of life.

Reflect

In Phil 4:8, Paul tells the Philippians to meditate on these things, and in 4:9 he tells them again to 'put into practice'. Routines are developed through practice; repeating behaviors over and over again. What behaviors is the Holy Spirit leading you to keep practicing over and over again?

_____

_____

_____

_____

_____

Reflect on some good routines that you currently practice. Why are they so important to you?

_____

_____

_____

_____

_____

Think about what throws you off your routine(s), such as vacations or birthdays. What can you do the next time to help you maintain your routine?

_____

_____

_____

_____

_____

Pray

Lord, I thank You that You have given me the ability to move my body each day. I choose to exercise as a form of worship. I will no longer see it as punishment, but as a celebration of my love for You. Thank You for changing me from the inside out so that I can see things differently—so I can start to see exercise differently. It will no longer be something I dread but rather something I look forward to. I'm excited for the day when exercise will become as natural for me as brushing my teeth! In Jesus' Name, Amen.

My Prayer

_____

_____

_____

_____

_____

_____

_____

_____

_____

_____

Additional Study Scriptures

*"Finally, brethren, whatever things are true, whatever things
are noble, whatever things are just, whatever things are pure,
whatever things are lovely, whatever things are of good
report, if there is any virtue and if there is anything
praiseworthy—meditate on these things."*
(Philippians 4:8 NKJV)

*"Teach them the statutes and laws,
and show them the way to live and the work they must do."*
(Exodus 18:20 BSB)

*"Teach me Your way, O LORD,
and lead me on a level path,
because of my oppressors."*
(Psalm 27:11 BSB)

Day 19:

Rise Up and Reward Yourself

Scripture Reflection

> *"No discipline seems pleasant at the time, but painful.*
> *Later on, however, it produces a harvest of righteousness*
> *and peace for those who have been trained by it."*
> (Hebrews 12:11 NIV)

Devotion

Today is Day 3 of understanding the habit loop.

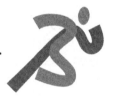

To recap:

Habits are formed by a 1. cue (seeing your **gym bag** at the door), which triggers 2. a routine (exercise), which is followed by 3. a reward.

It's reward that leads you to repeat the behavior the next time you experience the cue. This is the neurological loop that governs every habit (aka the habit loop.)

Rewards are critical in developing habits. We can easily see that in all our bad habits. We eat sweets because of the reward of the feeling it gives us.

Thankfully, rewards also work to form good habits like exercise. The good news is that exercise comes with a natural built-in reward—endorphins. When you exercise your body releases chemicals called endorphins, which is a chemical (like morphine) that makes you feel good. This takes a while to kick-in initially, so you will need to choose other things that motivate you.

The Bible tells us that we may not like the initial feeling of disciplining ourselves or being disciplined, but we will enjoy the rewards it provides us if we allow it to be our training ground. The same holds true for exercise. I don't know anyone who's ever said "I regret working out" ...have you?

It's the discipline it takes to get out of bed, put on your clothes, get off the couch, or just start. That's the hard part, but once you do the benefits and rewards are there.

Give yourself the best chance to maintain your exercise habit by choosing rewards that will keep you motivated and engaged. Keep them relevant and choose something that will actually make you feel good.

Tips on choosing rewards:

- Rewards are very individual, and they depend on your personality. Choose what will work for you:

- Offer thanksgiving and praise to God for your ability to exercise.

- Give yourself a check-mark on a calendar after a workout.

- Enjoy a relaxing cup of tea or coffee after your workout.

- Use a special body wash or lotion after your workout.

- Check it off on your calendar and reward yourself when you accumulate a certain number of points.

- Listen to your favorite songs during or after your workout.

- Listen to an audiobook or worship music.

- If it motivates you, take post-workout selfies and share them with your friends for encouragement.

- Say a prayer after every workout.

- Make your exercise time a time to talk to God.

- Splurge on some new exercise gear.

- Review your values. If you can align your values, it will also motivate you to stick to your exercise program. (See my book *Breakthrough* online course, weightlossgodsway.com/breakthrough, for lessons on your values.)

Reflect

What rewards have worked, and which ones have not worked in the past?

_____

_____

_____

_____

_____

What is the difference in how you feel before and after you exercise?

_____
_____
_____
_____
_____

Study Hebrews 12:11. What harvests (rewards) will you experience as you develop the habit of exercising consistently?

_____
_____
_____
_____
_____

Pray

Lord, I thank You that I am learning to treat myself with love and kindness. I'm learning how to practice self-care so that I can continue to bring glory to You. As exercise begins to become a daily habit and routine for me I'm so grateful for every opportunity I have to bring You glory. I give You all the thanks and praise for changing me from the inside out, for teaching me new healthy habits, and for reminding me that my body is Your temple. In Jesus' Name I pray. Amen.

My Prayer

_____
_____
_____
_____
_____
_____
_____
_____
_____
_____
_____
_____

Additional Study Scriptures

"And let us not grow weary of doing good,
for in due season we will reap, if we do not give up."
(Gal 6:9 NIV)

"But those who wait upon the LORD will renew their
strength; they will mount up with wings like eagles;
they will run and not grow weary; they will walk and not
faint." (Isaiah 40:31 ESV)

Day 20:

Rise Up and Master Your Mornings

Scripture Reflection

*"Let the morning bring me word of your unfailing love,
for I have put my trust in you. Show me the way I should go,
for to you I entrust my life."* (Psalm 143:8 NIV)

Devotion

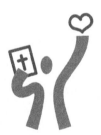

Now that you understand the habit loop,
let's apply it to your mornings.

Why mornings?

If you want to master good habits, you must take charge of
your mornings.

If you want to live a spirit-filled, productive day where you
feel alive, energized and flowing in your giftings, you must
'own your mornings'.

Mornings are the most important time of the day, because
they set the tone for the entire day. The start of each new day is

like a fresh opportunity to start over. It's like hitting the reset button (Lam. 3:23).

You can't roll out of bed at the last minute and wing it through the day.

Here's a simple morning routine that will help you maximize your day.

1. Set an alarm and wake up at the same time each day. Don't hit the snooze button (if you must, then no more than once).

2. Drink water (or lemon water). Drinking water is a way of turning on all your body systems. It's like flipping the 'on' switch in your body. It fires up your metabolism, your brain, and your digestive system. The lemon gives you a dose of vitamin C, revs up your metabolism, and is reported to decrease inflammation and joint pain.

3. Get into the Word. The Psalmist knew that walking with God first thing in the morning was foundational (Ps. 143:8). Isaiah also wrote that the Lord "wakens me morning by morning, wakens my ear to listen like one being instructed." (Is. 50:4)

It's God's Word that will set the course for the day. Without spending time in the Word it's so easy to get caught up in your agenda, your needs, and your wants. Even with our best attempts at planning, it will never come close to what God has in store for us each and every day. Be still and listen to what He telling you that is specific for each day. Approach Him with expectation and openness.

4. Plan your day. If you have not already planned it out the night before, spend a few minutes and be intentional about your

day. Did you plan in periods for rest? Have you thought about what you will be eating? What time will your day end? Notice that this follows prayer.

5. Exercise. This is ideal in the morning, but if your schedule does not permit then do it whenever time permits. Know that if making time for exercise is difficult for you, the later in the day you plan it the easier it will be to put other things in its place.

Reflect

Select one of the morning habits and then write out a cue and a reward that will help you to develop the habit so you can master it.

_____

_____

_____

_____

_____

What is the biggest challenge you have with "owning your mornings"?

_____

_____

_____

_____

_____

If you're not already doing it consistently, what would it take to begin exercising consistently each morning? What time would you have to wake up? What time would you have to go to bed?

_____
_____
_____
_____
_____

Pray

Heavenly Father, I thank You that your mercies are renewed every morning. When my heart is overwhelmed, You lead me back to You and it is there that I find rest and peace. When I feel like I'm stuck, remind me that I am never alone because You are always with me. Remind me that You always go before me and strengthen me. I thank You for giving me clarity in the midst of the difficulties, trials, and temptations. I thank You that I only need to keep my eyes and my mind fixed on You and it is there that I will find focus, strength, clarity, and peace for this journey. Restore my morning routine. Let me wake up each day with You on my mind. Let me seek You first thing each day and let the rest of my day be blessed and ordered, as a result of giving You the first fruits of my day.

My Prayer

_____
_____
_____
_____
_____
_____
_____
_____

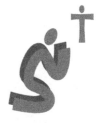

Additional Study Scriptures

"Satisfy us in the morning with your steadfast love,
that we may rejoice and be glad all our days."
(Psalm 90:14 ESV)

"And rising very early in the morning, while it was still dark,
he departed and went out to a desolate place,
and there he prayed." (Mark 1:35 ESV)

"O Lord, in the morning you hear my voice;
in the morning I prepare a sacrifice for you and watch."
(Psalm 5:3 ESV)

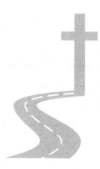

Day 21:

Week 3 Reflections

Scripture Reference

*"Give thanks in all circumstances;
for this is the will of God in Christ Jesus for you."*
(1 Thessalonians 5:18 ESV)

1. Recap– This week...

What did you learn about your body and how it relates to exercise over the past week?

_____
_____
_____
_____

2. Reflect

Journal what the Holy Spirit is showing you so far. How will this new habit help you align with your word for the year?

_____
_____
_____
_____

3. Pray

Commit your week to the Lord. Rest in Him and allow Him to give you the spirit of self-control and discipline.

_____

_____

_____

_____

_____

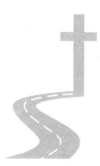

Day 22:

Rise Up and Keep it Simple

Scripture Reflection

"For an angel went down at a certain season into the pool, and troubled the water: whosoever then first after the troubling of the water stepped in was made whole of whatsoever disease he had." (John 5:4 NIV)

Devotion

Let's circle back to the sick man at Bethesda... Why was the man waiting at the pool?

The story goes that, one day, an angel would appear at the pool of Bethesda and stir up the water, and whoever was fast enough and 'lucky' enough to be the first in the water would receive their healing.

Not great odds for a paralyzed man, especially one with no friends to help him into the water!!

Before we judge him too harshly, let's ask ourselves how often we've hoped for miracles, believed the ads on TV, or tried gimmicks and fads to help us reach our goals. What great odds have you gone through to get 'instant' healing? Like the infirm man, the myths and miracles never panned out. The result was lots of wasted time and energy.

Yet, in an instant, Jesus healed him. No stirring water, no angel appearing, no competition. Just one encounter with Jesus.

Could it be that simple?

Jesus tells us that "Whoever drinks of the water that I will give him will never be thirsty again. The water that I will give him will become in him a spring of water welling up to eternal life." (John 4:14 ESV)

Don't know about you, but I'll choose the water that Jesus gives any day!

Beloved, know that there are no shortcuts to anything God wants to do in your life. He wants to restore you and strengthen you.

Will you trust Him today?

Reflect

In the Bible, Daniel began to get worried when his prayers were delayed. How did God speak to his prayers?

_____

_____

_____

_____

_____

Make a list of all of the gimmicks, miracle cures, and potions you've tried to get in shape or lose weight. Now surrender them all to God. Have a conversation with Him to remind yourself that His ways are best.

_____

_____

_____

_____

_____

_____

What are you still waiting on in your own strength that God can cure in an instant? Give it to Him today.

_____

_____

_____

_____

_____

_____

Pray

Lord, I thank You that Your way is best. When I'm following You, I don't need to worry or wonder if I'm doing the right thing. I trust You and Your ways. Continue to minister to me on this journey, and remind me that it is only in Your strength that I can do what You've called me to do. In Your Holy Name I pray! Amen!

My Prayer

_____
_____
_____
_____
_____
_____
_____
_____
_____
_____

Additional Study Scriptures

*"...but whoever drinks of the water that I will give him will
never be thirsty again. The water that I will give him will
become in him a spring of water welling up to eternal life."*
(John 4:14 ESV)

*"'Do not be afraid, Daniel,' he said, 'for from the first day
that you purposed to understand and to humble yourself
before your God, your words were heard, and I have come in
response to them'."* (Daniel 10:13 NIV)

*"But they that wait upon the Lord shall renew their strength;
they shall mount up with wings as eagles; they shall run,
and not be weary; and they shall walk, and not faint."*
(Isaiah 40:31 KJV)

Day 23:

Rise Up and Stop Making Excuses

Scripture Reflection

"Sir," the invalid replied, "I have no one to help me into the pool when the water is stirred. While I am trying to get in, someone else goes down ahead of me." (John 5:7 NIV)

Devotion

When Jesus asked the man if he wanted to be well, instead of saying 'yes' he told Jesus about his current bleak circumstances. He told Him why he probably would not be able to get well. Wouldn't you think that he would be saying, 'HECK, YES!!!'

But we can only surmise that he had grown so tired and so weary that where he once might have seen possibility, he now only saw pain. Where he once saw healing, he only saw heartbreak. So his only logical response now was to give reasons for why what he wanted was no longer possible.

Like him, excuses can become our automatic responses, our new normal, instead of holding on to our hope, promise, or expectation. **Excuses** justify why what we want is not possible.

Expectations declare what is possible when they are aligned with God's plans for us.

Why are we such excuse-making machines?

"I didn't work out today because I didn't have enough time."

"I'm not going to walk today because it's too cold outside."

"I want to exercise but I don't have the motivation."

It's so much easier to make excuses than it is to take responsibility and do whatever it takes to achieve our desired result. Excuses protect us from the fear of failure. It's not our fault—it's because we have no one to help us, because of the weather, or because of our time constraints. At the end of the day, the responsibility falls on our shoulders.

Thank goodness the Lord sees past our excuses, and will call us to take action in spite of them.

Know and believe that if God called you to it He will bring you through it. Trust that He will equip you and give you the strength you need to accomplish your tasks.

Reflect

Why do you make excuses instead of exercising? What do you feel is behind it? Pray about everything that comes up.

_____

_____

_____

The man had very legitimate reasons for why he had been there for so long. You probably do, too. Whether they are legitimate or a form of excuse-making, they still will not get you the results you desire. Distinguish between legitimate reasons vs. excuse-making, and get clear if there is a difference in God's eyes. In other words, can God still work in either situation?

Select a Scripture that you will recite and declare the next time you hear yourself making an excuse for why you cannot exercise.

Pray

Dear Lord, I have made excuses long enough. I want to get well! Show me what excuses are holding me back from glorifying You in my body, even the ones I hold subconsciously. You have empowered me with Your Holy Spirit. I claim that power and take 100% responsibility for my thoughts and actions. I will be active every day. In Your Holy Name, Amen.

My Prayer

_____
_____
_____
_____
_____
_____
_____
_____
_____
_____

Additional Study Scriptures

"I can do all things through Christ who strengthens me."
(Philippians 4:13)

"Arise, for it is your task, and we are with you;
be strong and do it." (Ezra 10:4)

"For each will have to bear his own load.
One who is taught the word must share all good things with
the one who teaches. Do not be deceived: God is not mocked,
for whatever one sows, that will he also reap. For the one
who sows to his own flesh will from the flesh reap corruption,
but the one who sows to the Spirit will from the Spirit reap
eternal life. And let us not grow weary of doing good, for in
due season we will reap, if we do not give up."
(Galatians 6:5-18)

Day 24:

Rise Up to Your Identity in Christ

Scripture Reflection

"When Jesus saw him lying there and learned that he had been in this condition for a long time, he asked him, 'Do you want to get well?'" (John 5:6 NIV)

Devotion

If you've been in a cycle of behavior for a long period of time, that behavior inevitably becomes a part of your identity.

These identities can bring productive blessings and prosperity to your life if the behaviors are healthy and productive, but the opposite is also true. Unhealthy cycles can produce unhealthy, self-defeating identities that leave us feeling void of life and powerless.

We see this cycle played out with the paralytic man. He had been in this condition for so long that his infirmity had become his identity. It's why he could not be made well.

It became his (legitimate) excuse for why he could not move forward in his life.

If we're not careful, we can also make the same mistake. Don't let your setbacks, challenges, or limitations define you.

If you're sick and tired of being sick and tired, and you are really ready to get well, then it's time to reclaim your life. Rise up and take small steps of faith every day.

Imagine what your life would look like if you were not stopped by your patterns of thinking and beliefs. For many that thought can be overwhelming, because it's a complete break from the life they've always known.

Imagine if you let go of all of the emotions and feelings that keep you bound.

You are not your illness, you are not your infirmity, you are not your weight or your body. You are not your bad habits. You are not your disappointments. You are not your limiting beliefs. You are a child of the King. You are who God says you are, and you can do what God says you can do!

Reflect

How would your life look different if you no longer held on to the belief or limitation that keeps you from exercising consistently?

_____

_____

_____

_____

_____

What would your response be if Jesus asked you if you want to get well? Could you say a resounding yes without any reservations or doubts. Give your doubts to Him if any come up.

_____

_____

_____

_____

_____

_____

Write out a long list of who you are in Christ. What is your true identity?

_____

_____

_____

_____

_____

_____

Pray

Lord, I thank You that my identity is in You. I am who You say I am and I can do all that You say that I can do. When I look in the mirror, I see that I am fearfully and wonderfully made—created in Your image. In Your Name, I pray. Amen!

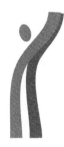

My Prayer

_____
_____
_____
_____
_____
_____
_____
_____
_____
_____

Additional Study Scriptures

*"The thief cometh not but for to steal, and to kill,
and to destroy: I am come that they might have life,
and that they might have it more abundantly."*
(John 10:10 KJV)

*"Therefore if any man be in Christ,
he is a new creature:
old things are passed away;
behold, all things are become new."*
(2 Corinthians 5:17)

*"But you are a chosen people, a royal priesthood,
a holy nation, God's special possession, that you may declare
the praises of him who called you out of darkness into his
wonderful light."* (1 Peter 2:9 NIV)

Day 25:
Rise Up and Manage Your Energy Levels

Scripture Reflection

> *"But David pursued, he and four hundred men, for two hundred who were too exhausted to cross the brook Besor remained behind."* (1 Samuel 30:10 NASB)

Devotion

When you're tired or drained, the last thing you want to do is exercise.

And there are probably some days when you would exercise if only you had the energy to do so. Unfortunately, all your great intentions and desires won't manifest if you're sleep-deprived, mentally drained, amped up on coffee, or lethargic from eating unhealthy foods.

But when you start effectively managing your overall energy levels, you will feel more inspired and encouraged to stay active.

In 1 Samuel 30:10, David's men were too exhausted to cross the valley. They were emotionally and mentally exhausted with grief at the capture of their wives (v 4), followed by physical exhaustion from trying to pursue their enemies. Two hundred of the 600 men finally wore out.

Wow, talk about a metaphor for life sometimes!

We can get so emotionally, mentally, and physically exhausted that we simply don't have the strength to make it through our valleys.

The secret is to equip ourselves for the long game so that we endure. Beyond this challenge, you need to keep going. This requires maximizing your energy spiritually, physically, and mentally.

Spiritually

Psalm 23:4 assures us that we can make it through the valleys when we cling to the truth that the Lord truly is our shepherd who guides us.

Physically

God created our bodies to store enough energy to get us through the day. But we then need to rest in order to recharge. Eating nutritious foods and getting plenty of rest are two important components in maintaining high energy levels.

Mentally

Mental fatigue will cause us to make poor choices. This is when we usually choose foods that will hurt us instead of healing us. It will cause us to put our immediate, temporal needs and wants before what's best for us in the long run. In the story of Jacob and Esau, we see how Esau's exhaustion led him to make a rash decision that would have eternal consequences (Genesis 25:29). Check your spiritual, physical, and mental energy. Which one do you need to maximize to allow you to remain active?

Reflect

What robs your energy? What will you do to reclaim it?

_____

_____

_____

_____

_____

What fills your tank and energizes you? How can you add more of it to your life?

_____

_____

_____

_____

_____

Think of your most productive, most rewarding, and most fun workouts or exercise sessions you've ever had. What contributed to it?

_____

_____

_____

_____

_____

Pray

Lord, I thank You for strengthening me during the difficult journeys. I understand that this is a marathon and not a sprint, and that I must gird myself up spiritually, mentally, and physically. Help me to maximize my energy so I don't quit before the finish line. I need Your strength to run this race with endurance. I need Your encouragement each and every day. I need You to help me move past my immediate needs. I keep satisfying my flesh, when it's my desire to live by Your Spirit so that I'm not constantly giving in to the desires of my flesh. I thank You for boundless energy that strengthens my witness and draws others to You. In Your Holy Name I pray. Amen!

My Prayer

_____

_____

_____

_____

_____

_____

_____

_____

_____

Additional Study Scriptures

> *"And do not get drunk with wine, for that is dissipation, but be filled with the Spirit."* (Ephesians 5:18 NASB)

"May God himself, the God of peace, sanctify you through and through. May your whole spirit, soul and body be kept blameless at the coming of our Lord Jesus Christ."
(1 Thes 5:23 NIV)

"For the word of God is quick, and powerful, and sharper than any two-edged sword, piercing even to the dividing asunder of soul and spirit, and of the joints and marrow, and is a discerner of the thoughts and intents of the heart."
(Hebrews 4:12 KJV)

Day 26:
Rise Up to Physical And Spiritual Renewal

Scripture Reflection

> *"Afterward Jesus found him in the temple and said to him, 'Behold, you have become well; do not sin anymore, so that nothing worse happens to you'."* (John 5:14 NIV)

Devotion

After healing the man at the pool at Bethesda physically Jesus runs into him in the temple, and after acknowledging his physical healing (*you have become well,*) speaks to his spiritual health by offering him a very stern rebuke. He says, *"do not sin anymore, so that nothing worse happens to you."*

Imagine telling someone who was infirm for most of his adult life that he would suffer a fate worse than that. What could be worse? Sin. Jesus tells him (and, as an extension, us) that sin can be even more debilitating. The effects of sin are worse bondage than being physically impaired. As much as you're working on your physical bodies, be sure to give more attention to your spiritual life.

Although you are here to build the habit of consistent exercise into your life, your first priority is to your spiritual health. Without being spiritually healthy you will continue to frustrate yourself, circling around the same mountain again. So take the time today to refuse to keep on sinning—whatever that looks like for you.

Commit to rooting out all conscious sin from your life. Don't settle for accepting sin as part of our human nature, and do your best to live according to the Spirit.

"Therefore, dear brothers and sisters, you have no obligation to do what your sinful nature urges you to do. For if you live by its dictates, you will die. But if through the power of the Spirit you put to death the deeds of your sinful nature, you will live." (Romans 8:12-13)

Paul also reminds us that physical exercise is of some value, but the real value comes from living a Godly life.

Once this challenge is over, continue to focus your attention on your spiritual health even more so than your physical health.

Reflect

Reflect on how much time you spend focused on self (in a negative way). Whether it's self-loathing or self-indulging, be honest (and non-judgmental) and transparent to God and let Him know that your desire is to fix your eyes on Him and not on self.

_____

_____

_____

When do you get most hyper-focused on self? Are you bored, tired, frustrated, or angry? The next time you find yourself focusing on your physical self, offer a prayer to God and thank Him for creating you so fearfully and wonderfully. Shift your focus to the Lord instead of self.

Reflect about your past attempts at getting more active or losing weight. How many times did you achieve your goal, only to revert to old habits. Like Jesus reminding the man that, even though he had become well, he was not to return to his old ways, heed the same advice as you also get well. Journal what the Holy Spirit is saying to you.

Pray

Lord, I thank You that You are concerned with my entire being. My body, soul, and spirit. I thank You for creating me as a tripartite being. My commitment is to live by Your Spirit so I will not give in to my sinful nature. I commit to rooting out all sin from my life, in Your Name. Amen!

My Prayer

_____

_____

_____

_____

_____

_____

_____

_____

_____

_____

Additional Study Scriptures

"For physical training is of some value, but godliness has value for all things, holding promise for both the present life and the life to come." (1 Timothy 4:8 NIV)

"But seek first the kingdom of God and His righteousness, and all these things will be added unto you." (Matthew 6:33 ESV)

"And Samuel said, 'Hath the LORD as great delight in burnt offerings and sacrifices, as in obeying the voice of the LORD? Behold, to obey is better than sacrifice, and to hearken than the fat of rams'." (1 Samuel 15:22 KJV)

Day 27:

Rise Up and Maintain Your Momentum

Scripture Reflection

> *"And let steadfastness have its full effect, that you may be perfect and complete, lacking in nothing. If any of you lacks wisdom, let him ask God, who gives generously to all without reproach, and it will be given him."* (James 1:4-5 ESV)

Devotion

I pray that this devotional and challenge has set the foundation for some great spiritual and physical habits that you will continue to practice for the rest of your life.

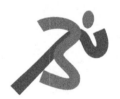

Let's wrap up these devotional reviewing habits. The upside of developing good habits is that they become routine. The downside of developing good habits is... that they become routine.

As great as habits and routines are, they can lead to boredom and stagnation if we don't keep things fresh. But isn't this what we wanted? To make healthy eating, exercise, and being led by the Spirit all routine so that they became automatic and habitual?

Yes, but even good habits also have a downside. It's only natural that when you do the same thing over and over again, you can lose the excitement, purpose, and even the desire to keep going.

James 1:4-5 not only tells us why we should maintain momentum as we grow, but tells us how we are to do it. He says that remaining steadfast will grow and mature us. He also says that we are to seek God to continue to teach us how to keep moving forward.

If it has not already started happening, it will. As you start to grow complacent or lose momentum, remember to pray and ask God for wisdom to help you endure. It says that God will generously provide it. We can ask for God's wisdom to guide our choices and decisions, to help us to understand the process, and to see this journey from His perspective.

Here's a short list of ways to maintain momentum. Pray and ask the Holy Spirit to show you how you can maintain your momentum throughout this journey.

- Create some short-term rewards and incentives.

- Never lose sight of the deeper purpose of being healthy—remember your 'Why'.

- Remind yourself of God's promises.

- Regular check-ins on your progress.

- Change up the routine—add some variety to your meals and workouts.

- Build in fun.

- Keep a gratitude journal.

- Practice mindfulness.

- Review your goals regularly.

- Build in accountability.

Reflect

Where are you in need of wisdom on this journey? Write out a prayer to God, asking Him to generously give it to you.

_____

_____

_____

_____

_____

_____

_____

In the last 27 days, did you become complacent or lose momentum? Try to recall the circumstances that led to it and write out what you can do in the future when it happens again.

_____

_____

_____

_____

_____

_____

_____

Make a list of tools that you use when you grow weary, then write out a short prayer or declaration that you will recite or confess.

_____

_____

_____

_____

_____

Pray

Lord, I will continue to seek Your best for me every day. In the highs and lows, I will never stop pursuing You. I will never stop making time for You. I will never stop submitting my plans and purposes to You. Help me to keep the zeal. Help me to remain steadfast. I rebuke the spirit of boredom and complacency. I find my strength and momentum in You so that I can continue on each day. You are my North Star, my guiding light that keeps me motivated. If I ever lose momentum or motivation, that's my cue to come back in alignment with You. Thank You for loving me so much that You will never let me wander away from You. In Jesus' Name, Amen.

My Prayer

_____

_____

_____

_____

_____

_____

_____

Additional Study Scriptures

"Let us not become weary in doing good, for at the proper time we will reap a harvest if we do not give up."
(Galatians 6:9 NIV)

"Those who sow in tears will reap with shouts of joy."
(Psalms 126:5 NIV)

"Therefore, my beloved brethren, be ye steadfast, unmovable, always abounding in the work of the Lord, forasmuch as ye know that your labor is not in vain in the Lord." (1 Corinthians 15:58 NIV)

Day 28:

Putting it all together

Congratulations on completing the Get Active, God's Way devotional & challenge!

Today, take time to reflect on the entire month, paying special attention to your successes and your challenges.

1. Recap

Review your progress from over the month.

1. Review your starting weight and ending weight.

2. How many days did you practice getting active? Is there room for growth?

3. What were some of your successes?

4. What were some of your challenges?

2. Reflect

What did the Holy Spirit reveal to you this week and during this entire month? Reflect on your word and verse for the year (if applicable). How was it manifested this month?

3. Pray

Thank God for what He has shown you, and commit the coming month to Him. Ask Him to help you commit to the practice of being active.

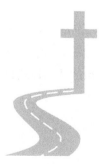

THANK YOU

Thank you for being motivated, courageous, inquisitive, and committed to go deeper into your health journey and uncover the missing piece—Christ!

I pray that these principles have been as much of a blessing to you as they have been for me and the hundreds of thousands of women around the world who have experienced what it means to include God in their health and weight-releasing journey.

If you've been blessed by this book, then please don't keep it a secret!

There are millions of women who need to hear this message. Please take a moment to leave an honest book review so more people can discover this book as well.

This book has laid out a great foundation for you, but there's so much more for you to discover. Please keep in touch with me so that you can stay in this conversation and continue to make your health a priority, God's way. Plus I'll send you a free copy of my 3 *Steps to Overcoming Emotional Eating* guide when you enroll for my weekly devotional message on successful weight loss, God's way.

cathymorenzie.com

Answers About Exercise

Frequently Asked Questions About Exercise

I've had the privilege of being a personal trainer for over 35 years, and during that time I've been asked hundreds if not thousands of questions. Fortunately most of the questions have been similar, so this section of the book will answer the most asked questions.

1. Question: *What's the best exercise to lose fat around my midsection?*

To answer this question effectively, two principles have to be addressed individually. 1. Best way to lose fat. 2. Fat around the midsection.

The best and only way to lose fat (short of liposuction) is to burn it off through activity. When you burn more calories (through activity) than you consume (through food) then you will lose weight. The best way to lose weight is with a combination of aerobic activity and strength training. Strength training is important because it will preserve your muscles, whereas, if you only do aerobic exercise, you will lose both fat and muscle.

Now, as far as losing weight about your mid-section. Unfortunately, you don't get to pick where you will lose fat. Fat loss usually is burned from the last place where you put on the weight. Last on, first off, and vice versa, so if you've always struggled with carrying excess weight in your midsection, working out might not change your proportions. You will just have less fat everywhere.

2. Question: Do I need to stretch before I work out?

Stretching will help to improve your flexibility and decrease your risk of injury; however, stretching is best performed after your workout. Stretching 'cold' muscles can actually increase your chance of injury. Prior to working out perform your activity at a lower intensity, and that should be sufficient to warm up your body.

3. Question: What are the best exercises for weight loss?

Similar to question #1, the best exercises to effectively lose fat are a combination of aerobic exercises (walking, running, swimming, cycling) with muscular strengthening exercises to maintain muscle strength. The more muscle mass you have the more fat you will burn, so don't be afraid to add weight training to your aerobic workouts to maximize your weight loss. Secondly, the best exercises for you are the ones that you enjoy. If you don't enjoy it then there's a higher chance that you will quit, so be sure to choose something fun.

4. Question: What do I do if I don't like to exercise?

Exercise is not everyone's cup of tea, but there are some things that you can do to change the way you feel about it, starting with making exercise fit in with your personality. Are you an introvert? Try swimming laps in a pool. Social butterfly? Try a Zumba or aqua-fit class. Competitive? Register and begin training for a race. Love the outdoors? Hiking is a great form of exercise. If you're easily bored, then continue to vary your routine. Create a list of 5-10 different things you like and change them frequently. Many of us have been forced to believe that exercise should look and feel a certain way in order to be effective. This is simply not true. Find what works for you and do it.

5. Question: How long do I need to work out to get results?

If you're new to exercise, start with about 15 minutes. Results will be minimal, but what's important is to begin to develop the habit.

6. Question: I always feel so hungry after exercise.
   Should I eat something?

It can seem like a catch-22. You start working out and your
appetite increases. What should you do? Eating more will ne-
gate all of the extra calories you burned off. If you find yourself
extra hungry after working out, first make sure you drink a lot
of water to make sure that it's not thirst you're experiencing
instead of hunger. Secondly, have a high protein meal after your
workout, which will help you to remain satisfied. Some examples include an egg, an apple with peanut butter, or a protein
shake.

7. Question: My muscles are so sore the day after. What
   should I do?

In the health and fitness world, sore muscles can be a good
thing once you understand the difference between muscle soreness due to working out effectively vs sore muscles due to injury.

If you're sore the day after or even a couple of days after,
you can perform some light activities and stretching. Listen to
your body and back off if it needs more recovery time. Muscle
soreness can kick up the same day, 24, 36, or even 48 hours
after a workout. If you're really sore, a nice Epsom salt bath can
also do the trick.

8. Question: How many days a week do I need to work out?

The number of days you exercise depends on the intensity and type of activities you are performing. You can perform light aerobic exercise such as walking, jogging, swimming, or cycling every day. Strength training, on the other hand, should be performed every other day depending on how intense your sessions are. It's best to work different muscles on alternate days so that your body can have a chance to rest. For example, if you perform squats or other leg exercises on Monday, then on Tuesday you can work your chest and arms and then return to legs on Wednesday, or even Thursday if they are still feeling tired or sore.

9. Question: I just can't seem to fit exercise into my day. What do I do?

Lack of time is the biggest reason that most people give for why they don't exercise, but the truth is that it's more of a priority issue than a time issue. Also, if you perceive that you will not be able to maintain your results, or if you're not sure what to do, then you will also procrastinate. As I highlighted in this book, start small and look for ways to incorporate small bouts of activity into your daily routine instead of trying to carve out an entire hour.

10. Question: Should I do cardio or weights first?

This depends on your goal. If your goal is weight loss then you should perform the cardio first, but if your main goal is to shape/tone/strengthen your muscles then you should perform the strength training portion first. Basically, in order to maximize your workout, do the most important type of exercise first because you will progressively fatigue the longer your workout session, so do the most important things first while your energy levels are highest.

11. Question: Do I need to take protein supplements if I'm working out?

Supplements are only recommended if you are working out with weights and are currently not consuming enough protein. Protein supplements are a good way to provide an additional source of protein without the additional calories, carbohydrates, and fat.

12. Question: I don't really sweat. How hard do I have to work out to get results?

Some people sweat more than others, so sweating is not a good indication of how hard you're actually working. The best way to determine how hard you should be exercising is to determine your target heart rate. To calculate your THR, you can use an on-line calculator like this one (https://www.active.com/fitness/calculators/heartrate) or you can use the following formula:

When exercising, select a target heart rate range between 50% - 85% of your heart rate reserve.

If you're just beginning start at the lower end of your range, and if you've been exercising for a while then you can push to the higher end.

To calculate:

- Subtract your age from 220 to get your maximum heart rate.

- Then determine your resting heart rate by counting how many times your heart beats per minute when you are at rest, such as first thing in the morning. For most people, it's somewhere between 60-90 beats per minute.

- Next, calculate your heart rate reserve (HRR) by sub-tracting your resting heart rate from your maximum heart rate.

- Then multiply your HRR by 0.6 (60%). Add your resting heart rate to this number.

- Lastly, multiply your HRR by 0.85 (85%). Add your resting heart rate to this number.

- The range between these two numbers is your aver-age target heart rate zone.

Example, if you're 50 years old and you want to figure out your target heart rate zone for moderate exercise using the HRR method, follow these steps:

- First, subtract your age of 50 from 220 to get 170 to determine your maximum heart rate.

- Next, find your resting heart rate first thing in the morning. Let's say it's 70 beats per minute. Then calculate your HRR by subtracting 70 (Resting Heart Rate from 170 (Maximum Heart Rate). This will give you a Heart Rate Reserve of 100.

- Then multiply 100 by 0.65 (65%) to get 65, then add your resting heart rate of 70 to get 135.

- Now multiply 100 by 0.75 (75%) to get 75, then add your resting heart rate of 70 to get 1145.

- So, your target heart rate zone for moderate exercise is 135–145 beats per minute.

So when you're exercising, stop briefly check your pulse for 15 seconds and ensure that it is in the range that you want to be working in. If it's lower than that you can push yourself a little harder, and if it's higher than that you can turn it down a bit.

13. Question: If I lift weights, will my muscles get bigger?

Bulging muscles is a fear that many women have when they begin lifting weights. However, most women's bodies are not designed to 'bulk up'. Lifting weight will sculpt, shape, and tone your body, but you will not bulk up unless you're taking steroids or lifting weights for several hours per day.

14. Question: I've been working out for three months and the scale has not budged. Am I doing something wrong?

Sometimes the scale not moving can be a good thing if you are exercising consistently, providing your diet has not changed. This could be an indication that you are building muscle mass, which is heavier than fat. If you're seeing other non-scale changes like decreased waist measurement or your clothes are fitting looser, then you should not worry too much.

However, if you don't see any of those changes either, there are a number of factors that affect weight loss, including stress, metabolism, and diet.

Stress

When you're stressed out your body releases cortisol, which preserves body mass. Meaning that your body holds on to weight as a survival mechanism. It's difficult to address weight loss without addressing your stress levels.

Metabolism

Next is your metabolism. Weight training boosts your metabolism. The more muscle you have on your body the higher your metabolism, as it takes more energy to burn muscle than fat since it's 3x more metabolically active than fat.

Food

If you're not releasing weight, check:

Are you consuming too many calories?

Are you consuming too few calories?

Are you consuming enough protein to preserve your lean muscle mass?

Are you consuming too much carbohydrates and sugar?

Are you consuming too much processed food or unhealthy fats?

Water

Are you drinking enough water each day? Your body needs water to process what you eat. Even if you're slightly dehydrated, your metabolism will slow down.

All of these factors will influence your weight release goals, so start here. And if there still is no change, you should consult your doctor.

15. Question: I've been doing the same workout for years. Do I need to change it?

It's important to vary your workouts, especially if you're no longer seeing results. Varying your workout can decrease your risk of injury. If your current workout overstresses some muscles while excluding others, varying your workout will give those muscles a chance to rest while building up neglected ones.

It will help you to break weight loss plateaus. Over time your body becomes more efficient, and the benefits you once experienced begin to decrease. This gives rise to fewer calories burned if you're doing aerobic workouts and less strengthening of the muscles if you're performing strength training workouts.

Changing your workouts will also keep you from getting bored, which will keep you motivated and increase your adherence to your goal. Boredom and complacency are a big reason why many people quit, so don't be afraid to change up your routine at least every 12 weeks or so.

16. Question: Do I need to keep working out this hard once I achieve my goal weight?

Hopefully once you've made exercise a habit you will want to continue working out. However, you will not have to work out as hard during maintenance as you did when you were working to achieve your goal. If your goal of working out was to release excess weight, in order to do that you needed to create a caloric deficit by burning more calories than you consumed. Once you achieve your goal weight, your new goal is to balance your calories consumed with your calories expended (burned).

17. *Question:* Is it better to work out on an empty stomach?

There are many pros and cons to working on an empty stomach, otherwise known as in a fasted state. There are two schools of thought on this topic. One side believes that it will help your body to burn more fat because your body will use the stored fat for energy instead of the food you've recently eaten, which will lead to higher levels of fat loss.

On the flip side, if you work out on an empty stomach you may not have as much energy during your workout, and it can even leave you feeling light-headed and nauseated. Give it a try and see how you feel. If you feel great after doing it then go for it, otherwise sample different light meals that you could have before your workout. Be sure that your meal is easy to digest and contains a combination of carbohydrates, fats, and proteins such as some almond butter on whole grain bread, a protein shake, or some oatmeal. Also, give yourself enough time for your food to digest before working out.

If you do choose to work out in a fasted state, be sure to drink a lot of water before and throughout the day and, as always, listen to your body.

18. *Question:* I always hear the expression, 'No pain, no gain'. Should I just push through minor aches and pains as I work out?

You may have heard the expression, 'no pain, no gain', but it's important to note that not all pain is beneficial. There's a place for 'feeling the burn' when it comes to working out, but it's important to be able to distinguish between good muscle fatigue and bad muscle fatigue or joint pain, or possibly injury.

When performing aerobic exercise, determine how hard you should be working by calculating your target heart rate. See question 12.

When performing muscular strength training, you want to select a weight where your muscles feel fatigued in your last couple of repetitions. The goal is to fatigue the muscle, so you will need to determine how many repetitions it will take before your muscles fatigue. The recommended number of repetitions to perform is between 10-15, but recognize that it is a very general rule. If you want to see more muscle growth, then lift heavier weights so that your muscles will fatigue with less repetitions. And if you just want to maintain your strength without seeing much change in the shape or size of the muscle, then you can perform higher repetitions and use lighter weights.

19. *Question:* I'm losing weight by eating less and exercising but my skin is getting saggy. What should I do?

If you've lost a significant amount of weight, your skin may have a difficult time snapping back to its original state, due to damaged collagen and elastin fibers in your skin. Sagging skin has a lot to do with genetics, so in some cases there's not a lot you can do. However, building muscle mass through weight training can definitely help to reduce the appearance of loose skin. Pilates is often recommended to tighten loose skin because of its focus on strengthening the core.

The likelihood of sagging skin is also prevalent more with rapid weight loss. So if you're on a weight loss program, gradual weight loss will also help to alleviate this problem.

I hope I answered your fitness question amongst these most popularly asked questions. If not, please do not hesitate to reach out to me at support@cathymorenzie.com.

May God continue to bless you on your journey!

Leader's Guide

Get Active, God's Way
Leader's Guide

"Therefore go and make disciples of all nations,
baptizing them in the name of the Father and of the
Son and of the Holy Spirit, and teaching them to obey
everything I have commanded you. And surely I am
with you always, to the very end of the age."
(Matt 19:20)

Thank you for answering the call to lead a group through the Get Active, God's Way 28-day challenge and devotional. Coming together as a group holds you accountable, and provides an opportunity to develop consistency within your faith. The best way to learn is to teach. We believe that as you lead others, you will also continue to grow in the Lord.

Healthy by Design ignites and mobilizes leaders who want to use their spiritual gifts and skills so that others can be transformed by the truth of God's Word.

Know that when you say 'yes' to ministering to others, you are changing and affecting not only their lives but also the lives of everyone they come into contact with. You will find that, as a leader, you will feel more connected with the devotionals as you take on a sense of ownership and responsibility and want to support your small group as much as possible.

You have the option of leading the challenge online or in an in-person group. As a leader, you must register your courses with us. Please register your group here:

https://www.cathymorenzie.com/become-a-bible-studyleader/

The 28-day challenge/devotional works best when participants work independently and follow up their independent study with leader-led small-group interaction, either in person or virtually.

As the group leader, your responsibility is to facilitate discussion and conversation and make sure that everyone gets the most out of the devotionals. You are not responsible for having

all the answers to people's questions or reteaching the content. That's what the devotional is for.

Your role is to guide the experience, encourage your group to go deeper into God's Word, cultivate an atmosphere of learning and growth amongst a body of believers, and answer any questions that the group may have.

Tips to get the most from the Small Groups Sessions

1. It's about God. Although we use biblical principles to guide us on how to address strongholds in our lives, remember that it's always about God. Your role as a leader is to always point everyone to the cross.

2. Partner up. Have your group choose an accountability partner to go through the devotional with. It's always more encouraging when you can connect with someone on a regular basis in addition to when you meet as a group.

3. Keep a journal. Encourage your group to use a supplemental journal. They can choose from an online journal like Penzu (penzu.com) or use old-school pen and paper. Either way, taking time to record your thoughts, feelings, inspirations, and directives from the Holy Spirit is a great way to maximize the experience.

4. Be consistent. Meet at the same time and location each week. This will help the group to organize their time and their schedules. Try to select a time that works best for everyone.

5. Plan ahead. Take time prior to the weekly study to think about how you will present the material. Think about a story or example that would add to the material.

Think about the most effective way to make use of the time.

6. Keep it intimate. Keep the small group small. I suggest a maximum of 12-15 people. This will create a more relaxed and transparent atmosphere so that people will feel safe to speak.

7. Be transparent. You can set the tone for the group by sharing your story. This will help people to feel safe and establish trust with them. When you speak, give personal examples and avoid phrases like 'some people' and 'Christians'.

8. Be professional. Always start and end the sessions on time. Communicate clearly if you see that you will be going overtime. Apologize and let them know how much you respect their time.

9. Bring lots of energy. Let your passion for studying God's Word be evident. Remember that your energy level will set the tone for the entire group, so bring it!

10. Pray. It might sound obvious, but make sure that prayer is an intricate part of the entire process. Pray at the beginning and end of every session. Feel free to call on others to lead the prayers. During the session, you can have one person pray for the entire group—have one person open and another close— ask for requests, or select someone. You can also encourage the group to pray for one another. Lastly, don't forget to pray during the time leading up to the session.

11. Keep it simple. If the sessions get too complicated, people will find reasons not to attend. If you plan to serve snacks, keep it simple and nutritious. Don't plan weekly potlucks that will require the group members to do too much work.

12. Be creative. Feel free to add music, props, or anything that you feel will add to the environment and facilitate learning.

13. Be comfortable. Make sure there is adequate comfortable seating for everyone. Check the temperature in the room. Alert everyone as to where the bathrooms are located.

Preliminary Preparation

Pray and seek the Holy Spirit on whether you should participate in this devotional.

Determine with your group how long you will meet each week, so you can plan your time accordingly. Most groups like to meet from 1-2 hours.

Promote the challenge and devotional through community announcements, social media, in your church bulletin, or simply call a few of your friends.

Send out an email to a list or send a message on social media announcing the upcoming study.

Prior to the first meeting, make sure that everyone purchases a copy of the devotional. Include a link where they can purchase it.

Have the group read Day 1 and be prepared to share their responses.

Suggested Group Plan

Because *Get Active, God's Way* is an independent devotional and challenge, the group discussion will incorporate a series of small discussions within the greater discussion. Feel free to customize the design to fit the needs of your group. The suggested plan is for a four-week session. Following is the breakdown.

A Four-Week Session Plan

Session 1

1. Welcome everyone to the session and open with prayer.

2. Share a bit about yourself. Then go around the room and have everyone introduce themselves. Have each person share what their current exercise regimen looks like.

What are the challenges and stresses they face? Are they consistent or sporadic? Do they walk or go to the gym?

3. Give an overview of the devotional and a brief overview of the *Get Active, God's Way* challenge and devotional. Read the Day 1 Devotional, 'Why Rise Up' and ask your group if they are ready to 'rise up'.

4. Housekeeping Items:

- format for the session
- confirm dates and times
- where bathrooms are
- rules for sharing
- commitment to confidentiality
- attendance each week
- snacks (have volunteers provide)

5. Offer suggestions to get the most out of the study.

Ask the group what level of challenge they will be partici-
pating in, and encourage them to complete them each day. Consider offering weekly incentives or prizes.

6. Stress the importance of trust and transparency.

7. Instruct the group to complete the six days before the
next session. Encourage them to carve out some time each day
to complete the devotions and to do their chosen level of activity.

8. Review the Day 1 devotion and ask the group to share their
responses.

Suggested Discussion Starters:

- What can you learn from the story that applies to
  your life?

- Why is it important for you to Rise Up in this season
  of your life?

- What stops you from developing a consistent exercise routine?

- What negative beliefs do you have about exercise
  that sabotages you?

- What difference would it make in your life if you began to see exercise as a form of worship?

- How is the Holy Spirit speaking to you?

9. Have the group read Week 2 for next week's session.

10. Close the session in prayer.

Session 2

1. Welcome the group.

2. Start with an opening prayer.

3. Ask the group what insights/breakthroughs/testimonials they encountered as a result of what the Holy Spirit has been showing them.

Suggested Discussion Starters (from Week 2):

- What baby steps can you take instead of trying to make big sweeping changes?

- What are some of the things that rob your time?

- Why did Jesus tell the man at the pool to take up his bed (mat)?

- How is God calling you to 'rise up' and look at your health differently?

- What difference will it make in your life when you trust in the Lord to help you get active instead of re-lying on your own strength?

4. Make a closing remark or statement to tie in the entire conversation.

5. Have the group read Week 3 for next week's session.

6. End with a closing prayer.

Session 3

1. Welcome the group.

2. Start with an opening prayer.

3. Ask the group what insights/breakthroughs/testimonials they encountered as a result of what the Holy Spirit has been showing them.

Suggested Discussion Starters (from Week 3):

- How can you make exercise a time of worship?

- Explain in your own words the habit loop.

- What are some of your cues that will trigger you to exercise?

- What throws you off your exercise routine?

- How will you 'reward' yourself?

- Why is it important to seek the Lord in the morning?

4. Have the group read Week 4 for next week's session.

5. End with a closing prayer.

Session 4

Think about how you will make the final session memorable. Maybe end with a group walk, do one of my exercise videos together, or give out little rewards to the group's commitment to exercise.

1. Welcome the group.

2. Start with an opening prayer.

3. Ask the group what insights/breakthroughs/testimonials they encountered as a result of what the Holy Spirit has been showing them.

Suggested Discussion Starters (from Week 4):

• What excuses do you make for not exercising?

• What would your response be if Jesus asked you if you want to get well?

• What fills your tank and energizes you? How can you add more of it to your life?

• Why did Jesus offer the man a stern rebuke after healing him (John 5:14)?

• How has your attitude towards exercise changed over the last few weeks?

• How has the Holy Spirit been speaking to you?

4. Wrap up the session with closing words/thoughts. Encourage the group to continue the great work that they've begun.

5. End the session with a closing prayer.

Thank you again for taking the time to lead your group. You are making a difference in the lives of others, and having an impact on the Kingdom of God.

Other Weight Loss God's Way Offerings

Weight Loss God's Way (weightlossgodsway.com) equips women to rely on God as their strength so they can live in freedom, joy, and peace. At the end of the day, that's what we really want. Let's be honest, if you've never achieved that mythical, elusive number on the scale, but were fully able to live a life of freedom, joy, and peace, would that be enough? I know for me the answer is a resounding YES!!!

We provide a multidimensional approach to releasing weight. It encompasses the whole person—spiritual, psychological, mental, nutritional, physical, and even hormonal! We believe that you must address the whole person—body, soul, and spirit. If you're looking for a program that just tells you what to eat and what exercises to do, this ain't it.

This program has helped thousands of women break free from all the roadblocks that have been hindering their weight loss success while discovering their identity in Christ.

Weight Loss God's Way offers a variety of free and paid courses and programs. They include the following:

A YouVersion Bible Studies:

A free basic introduction to Step 1 of the Weight Loss, God's Way program. To learn more, go to:

https://my.bible.com/reading-plans/4593-weight-loss-gods-way.com

Or from the YouVersion Bible App, click the bottom center, 'check-mark' button to open devotions, and search for Weight Loss God's Way or our other free devotionals:

Rest, Restore, and Rejuvenate

Praying for Your Health

The Weight Loss, God's Way Devotional Newsletter

Join the free Weight Loss, God's Way community and receive regular posts designed to help you align your weight loss with God's Word. You'll also receive a special bonus gift just for joining. To join the newsletter, sign up at:

cathymorenzie.com

The Membership Program

A done-for-you, step-by-step guide to our entire program. Dozens of bonus tools like group coaching calls, forums, and accountability groups. To become a Weight Loss, God's Way member, go to:

weightlossgodsway.com

Bible Studies for Churches and Small Groups

The membership program can also be experienced a la carte with a group of your friends or with your church. Take one of our three-to-six-week studies on a variety of health and weight-releasing topics. To learn more about starting a Bible study in your home or church, go to:

https://www.cathymorenzie.com/start-a-wlgw-group/

Books and Devotionals

You can find all of our Healthy by Design series of weight loss books here:

Christianweightlossbooks.com

Keynote Speaking

Want me to visit your hometown? Need a speaker for your annual conference or special event? My fun and practical approach to Weight Loss, God's Way will give your group clarity and focus to move toward their weight loss goals. To learn more or to book a speaking engagement, visit:

https://www.cathymorenzie.com/speaking/

Private Coaching

Prefer a more one-on-one approach? I have a few dedicated time slots available to coach you individually to help you fast-track your results. To learn more, go to:

https://www.cathymorenzie.com/coach-with-cathy/

Other Healthy by Design books by Cathy Morenzie:

The Breakthrough Method:
Your Guided Path to Weight Loss, God's Way

Weight Loss, God's Way:
The Proven 21-Day Weight Loss Devotional Bible Study

Weight Loss, God's Way:
Low-Carb Cookbook and 21-Day Meal Plan

Pray Powerfully, Lose Weight

Love God, Lose Weight

Healthy Eating, God's Way

Spirit-Filled and Sugar-Free

The Word on Weight Loss

Continue the **journey!**

Lose weight, God's way
in our *21-Day Intensive Course*
'The Breakthrough Method'

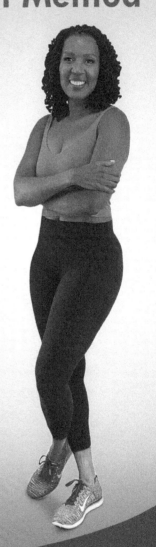

21 Daily Insights
and Videos from
Cathy Morenzie

21daysgodsway.com

About The Author

Cathy is a noted personal trainer, author, blogger and presenter, and has been a leader in the faith/fitness industry for over a decade. Her impact has influenced hundreds of thousands of people over the years to help them lose weight and develop positive attitudes about their bodies and fitness.

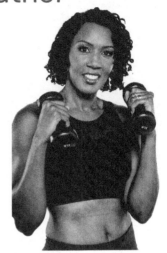

Over the years, she has seen some of the most powerful and faith-filled people struggle with their health and their weight.

Cathy Morenzie herself—a rational, disciplined, faith-filled personal trainer—struggled with her own weight, emotional eating, self-doubt, and low self-esteem. She tried to change just about everything about herself for much of her life, so she knows what it's like to feel stuck. Every insecurity, challenge, and negative emotion that she experienced has equipped her to help other people who face the same struggles—especially women.

With her Healthy by Design books and Weight Loss, God's Way programs, Cathy has helped thousands to learn to let go of their mental, emotional, and spiritual bonds that have kept them stuck, and instead rely on their Heavenly Father for true release from their fears, doubts, stress, and anxiety. She also teaches people how to eat a sustainable, nutritious diet, and find the motivation to exercise.

Learn more at www.cathymorenzie.com.

Follow Cathy at:
https://www.facebook.com/weightlossgodsway/
youtube.com/@CathyMorenzieWeightLossGodsWay
pinterest.com/cathymorenzie
instagram.com/cathy.morenzie

Made in the USA
Monee, IL
30 May 2024

59114507R00098

40 Women share inspiring stories of perseverance in spite of adversity and choose to walk through life with purpose, persistence, and awareness.

THE DECONSTRUCTING G.R.I.T. COLLECTION

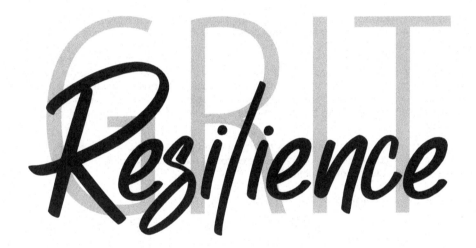

GRIT
Resilience

COMPILED BY
JENNIFER BARDOT

RESILIENCE - Deconstructing G.R.I.T. Collection
40 Women share inspiring stories of perseverance in spite of adversity
and choose to walk through life with purpose, persistence, and awareness
MDC Press

Published by **MDC Press**, St. Louis, MO
Copyright ©2023
All rights reserved.

Cover, Interior Design, and Project Management:
  Davis Creative Publishing Partners, CreativePublishingPartners.com
Writing Coach and Editor: Maria Rodgers O'Rourke

Compilation by Jennifer Bardot

Library of Congress Cataloging-in-Publication Data (Produced by Cassidy Cataloguing Services, Inc.)

Names: Bardot, Jennifer, compiler.
Title: Resilience the deconstructing G.R.I.T. collection / compiled by Jennifer Bardot.
Other titles: Resilience GRIT
Description: St. Louis, MO : MDC Press, [2023]
Identifiers: ISBN: 978-1-7371848-4-3 (paperback) | 978-1-7371848-5-0 (ebook) | LCCN: 2022923719
Subjects: LCSH: Resilience (Personality trait)--Literary collections. | Resilience (Personality trait)-- Anecdotes. | Self-actualization (Psychology) in women--Literary collections. | Self- actualization (Psychology) in women--Anecdotes. | Awareness--Literary collections. | Awareness--Anecdotes. | Perseverance (Ethics)--Literary collections. | Perseverance (Ethics)--Anecdotes. | LCGFT: Anecdotes.
Classification: LCC: BF698.35.R47 R48 2023 | DDC: 155.24--dc23

*I dedicate this book to all
who are committed each day
to living out their personal purpose
no matter what.*
–Jennifer Bardot

Surrendering

Thawing, like freezing
but more visible, happens in layers,
slowly as crystals melt, or suddenly
as clumps of snow collapse
off pine boughs. It can also be
disguised, subtle as black ice, or
symbolic, as
we recognize it's time to shed the fears
we used to stay alive, that shielded our
emerging, eager spirits. It will be hard.
If only we, like sycamores, could let our withered
bark peel off to gently bare abandoned dreams,
that still as death, somehow survived.
Lying in wait, an
impatient ego lures us with
the swooning, slumping,
threat of fresh abandonment,
a tempting ploy to keep us
trapped inside our paradox.

We hear our inner

voices, the ones that always caution us

to wait, but bolstered by awareness,

we detach ourselves from pain that

has become irrelevant, which

like stripping old paint, takes time. It is

a process, a project that has commenced

again and again,

each stage silenced by our first companions –

fear and doubt – formed to keep our little

selves and secrets safe. Now, we silence

them. You see, we've learned surrendering is

not the same as giving up or giving in.

It is assenting

to the deferred demise of useless attitudes

and vain conceits, a rebuttal

to the acts of insolence, a leaving off of

habits and addictions that will no longer

keep us from emerging, as we thaw.

– Cheryl Roberts